CANCER SURVIVOR'S NUTRITION & HEALTH GUIDE

Eating Well and Getting Better During and After Cancer Treatment

GENE SPILLER, PH.D., AND BONNIE BRUCE, DR.P.H., R.D.

PRIMA PUBLISHING

To the cancer survivors,
that this book may help them on their path
to complete recovery, strength, and lasting health.
Gene Spiller and Bonnie Bruce

Illustrations: John Richards

Library of Congress Cataloging-in-Publication Data

Spiller, Gene A.
  Cancer survivor's nutrition and health guide : eating well and getting better during and after cancer treament / by Gene Spiller and Bonnie Bruce.
        p. cm.
    Includes index.
    ISBN 0-7615-0581-4
      1. Cancer—Nutritional aspects.   2. Cancer—Diet therapy.   I. Bruce, Bonnie.
  II. Title.
  RC268.45.S65   1996
  616.99'40654—dc20   96-32749
                                                                  CIP

96 97 98 99 00 01 AA 10 9 8 7 6 5 4 3 2 1
Printed in the United States of America

HOW TO ORDER

Single copies may be ordered from Prima Publishing, P.O. Box 1260BK, Rocklin, CA 95677; telephone (916) 632-4400. Quantity discounts are also available. On your letterhead, include information concerning the intended use of the books and the number of books you wish to purchase.

Visit us online at http://www.primapublishing.com

Contents

Part Two
Recipes for Recovery and Protection from Future Illness

Acknowledgments

RECIPES FROM TWO KEY CONTRIBUTORS AND THE ADVICE of two dietitians, in addition to help from others, have been key in making this a useful book for the cancer survivor:

Monica Spiller is the author of many of the recipes in *Eat Your Way to Better Health* and *Nutrition Secrets of the Ancients*. She is the author of *The Barm Bakers' Book* and has taught classes for professional bakers at Mission College in California. Monica is actively engaged in developing recipes that utilize ancient ways of preparing whole, unrefined foods and is a consultant to bakers on whole grain breads. She is a consistent and inspiring supporter of the concept of unrefined foods.

Rowena Hubbard is a registered dietitian and the president of Food Resources in Sacramento, California, where she operates a test kitchen. She has contributed recipes to *Eat Your Way to Better Health* and is a coauthor of *Nutrition Secrets of the Ancients*. Rowena has done recipe development and editing work on a series of international recipes for a Spice Islands book series on foods and has contributed several sections to the Time-Life Book Series *Meals in Minutes*. She is also the coauthor of one of the first books on California cuisine, *California Cooks*. In addition, she has developed, edited, and published recipes for a wide range of clients and consumer magazines. Rowena is currently the food consultant of the *Napa Valley Record.* She is co-owner of a whole foods company, Classic Grains, which provides whole, natural food products to the food service industry.

Two dietitians have shared with us their clinical expertise about cancer patients during crucial stages of treatment and recovery: Diane Hester, MS, RD, CNSD, is the clinical nutrition manager and Tara Coghlin, MS, RD, is a clinical dietitian at the Stanford University Hospital Department of Nutrition and Food Services in Palo Alto, California.

Additional thanks to John Potter, M.D., head of the cancer prevention research program at the Hutchinson Cancer Research Center in Seattle, Washington, who places fruits and vegetables at the top of his list of foods that protect against cancer.

Rosemary Schmele has been invaluable in various stages of manuscript development and proofreading.

John Richards, a Menlo Park artist who created many of the illustrations in this book, divides his time between artwork and teaching environmental education to children at Hidden Villa Wilderness Preserve in Los Altos Hills, California.

We are also thankful to Georgia Hughes of Prima Publishing, who suggested to us this book and made possible its publication. Georgia has become more than an editor, she has become a friend. And Betsy Towner at Prima Publishing was invaluable in the final stages of editing and production.

Introduction

THIS BOOK IS FOR YOU, THE CANCER SURVIVOR. IT'S designed to help you get well and—just as important—to stay well and do all you can to prevent recurrence. Every day we learn more about health and disease, and we are finding that the foods best for disease prevention should also be our first choices during treatment and recovery. These foods may need to be specially prepared to make them easier to eat or gentler on a digestive system affected by therapy, but their essence is always the same.

Two key concepts at the forefront of nutrition have guided our writings: First, if a diet is to be optimal, it must be based on plant foods, with only limited amounts of selected animal products, such as lowfat or nonfat milk products. Second, the plant foods we choose should be as unrefined as possible, with all their natural goodness left undamaged. Both the path to recovery and the path to health maintenance must be paved with these principles. However, neither of these concepts will work if the food is not appealing, and so, our writings have also been guided by a third principle: namely, that whatever we cook must taste good.

You will find a program of eating laid out in this book that will provide ample nourishment and enjoyment in addition to helping you restore your energy, replenish and rebuild your body, and significantly protect against future cancer. The recipes are wholesome and simple, packed with building and protective nutrients. They include variations for special needs, such as low-fiber and easy-to-chew or -swallow meals, for periods when the effects of treatment result in low appetite and a weak digestive system.

All this should help you get back to a high energy level and to make you feel stronger. You'll feel that you are doing everything you can to maximize the benefits and minimize the aftereffects of cancer treatment. And, after the treatment is completed, you'll know you are doing your best to protect yourself from new cancers.

In this book, you will find ideas about how to overcome some of the aftereffects you may be experiencing, like nausea or the outright rejection of food. You'll find ideas on how you can entice yourself to eat when you have no appetite or are too tired to prepare something for yourself, and what foods you should eat if you have difficulty swallowing, a dry mouth, or bouts of diarrhea or constipation.

You will be able to use the information in this book immediately. The sooner you get started, the sooner you will be on the journey to replenishing your body, restoring your strength and health, and making the most beneficial changes in your diet to reduce your risks of disease recurrence and increase resistance to future illness. Our philosophy is based on scientific research and information from cancer survivors about what kinds of things worked for them. This book should bring about a new way of eating that the cancer survivor will find appealing and pleasurable, a way of eating that should be the foundation of your food choices for a lifetime of disease prevention.

Part One tells you the why and how of the path to recovery and health. Chapter 1, "The Path to Health," and chapter 2, "The Key Foods for Restoring and Maintaining Health," begin the journey by describing the foods that should be the foundation of healing, recovery, and protection for the cancer survivor. These two chapters bring to life the art of eating during treatment and recovery by exploring the links between good nutrition and nature's pharmacy of foods.

Chapter 3, "Herbs, Spices, Teas, and the Magic of Clustering," introduces ancient, little-discussed dimensions to healthy eating—things such as herbs and spices that have protective components. And it gives you a creative technique for seeing how your foods produce a synergy of effects that contribute to health, the technique of clustering. Chapter 4, "Putting It All Together," takes key superfoods and puts them into a unique and novel pyramid format (the Cancer Survivor's Pyramid) to meet the special eating needs of cancer survivors during different phases of treatment and recovery.

Chapter 5, "Handling Special Situations," is a very important chapter. If you do not have any problems during treatment you do not need to read it, or if you have a special problem, you may just want to read about that problem and how to handle it. It discusses strategies for taking care of many of the physical aftereffects of treatment, such as nausea and constipation. You'll find suggestions there on how to make changes in diet, ways of eating, and examples of menus to help you get the most out of your meals during these temporary difficult periods.

Chapter 6, "Beyond Food," is to remind you that there is more to recovery and later disease prevention than food. It covers some other things you should do, or should avoid, to heal and do the best you can to prevent cancer recurrence.

Part Two is the practical part of the book, with recipes for maximizing recovery and for protecting you against future illness.

Each one of us has a different background: The genes we have inherited from our parents, the way we have been fed as infants and children, and later, the way we have chosen to eat and drink. Add to all this previous exposure to environmental agents—such as smoke, pollution, radiation, to name a few—and the stage of your cancer when you began therapy, and the range of diversity becomes evident. You cannot undo your past and that past will to a great extent influence the success of the suggestions made in this book, but you can do the best you can to recover and then stay healthy. And remember that this book is not intended as a substitute for medical advice. Always consult your physician, registered dietitian, or another qualified health professional whenever you have a medical or nutritional concern.

PART ONE

Vital Information

Chapter 1

THE PATH TO HEALTH

PICTURE YOUR BODY AS A MARVELOUS MACHINE, SUCH as a fine car in need of major repairs. First of all, you need to do whatever major repairs need to be done; secondly, after the repairs are completed, you need to do some fine tuning. When all this is done and you are ready to use your now "healthy" machine, you need to do your best to keep it in super shape. This means you must use it properly, and give it the best possible fuel and other needed fluids to prevent it from needing repair again. And, if there is a weak link in the system, you must do all you can to protect it as you use it.

As a cancer survivor, you are, indeed, just like this automobile, and your body, the human body, is the most complex of all machines. Something went wrong, for whatever reason. Some powerful medicines, surgery, radiation, or whatever methods you have chosen to repair it with, have been used to treat the degenerated cells—the cancer cells, but at the same time, the treatment has caused some damage to other cells and organs in your body. This has led to weakness. Your resistance to infection is probably lower, and you are experiencing other problems such as poor appetite and a weaker digestive system. During this time, more than ever, you need energy, which means calories; you need proteins to build and rebuild damaged tissues, and you need all the possible protective nutrients that foods can provide. Most of all, you need to build up your overall health. The key to better health lies, just as with the car, with three basic things: The best possible care, fuel, and protective substances.

In this chapter, we will discuss the key factors for recovery, the need for energy and carbohydrates, proteins, fats, vitamins and minerals, fiber and phytochemicals, and water. *Remember: As you pursue better health, think of the three basic steps—first repair, second fine tuning, and third proper use and protection.*

THE KEY FACTORS FOR RECOVERY

The cancer survivor, more than anyone else, needs:

1. Calories, to supply essential energy. These are best obtained from *carbohydrate* foods as well as from *good fats.* The most desirable sources include whole grains and cereals, cooked dry beans, peas, lentils, fruits, vegetables, nuts and seeds, olive oil, and wheat germ oil.

2. Proteins, for building and rebuilding tissues in the body. Premier sources are, again, whole grains and cereals, cooked dry beans, peas, lentils, tofu, and nuts and seeds. Also included in this group are nonfat or low–fat milk, yogurt, cottage cheese, and ricotta cheese.

3. Protective compounds, to help ward off recurrence of cancer. There are thousands of protective compounds and they include *fiber, vitamins, minerals,* and that newly emerging family of plant compounds, which boasts hundreds of members, the *phytochemicals* ("phyto" means plant). Premier foods here include whole grains and cereals, cooked dry beans, peas, lentils, fruits, vegetables, nuts and seeds, and the good fats like extra virgin olive oil and wheat germ oil.

Just as important are food textures, form (liquid or solid), and appearance to entice and motivate you to eat. This means that, as you begin your journey on the path to healing and protecting, you need to stock the pantry with foods from nature's own pharmacy, foods that should be as close as possible to the way nature provided them, with all their goodness left intact.

Unfortunately, many common foods in the typical American diet have been refined, manipulated, overprocessed, and engineered to such a degree that sometimes few naturally occurring protective compounds are left. The refined, low plant food, high animal food American diet has been called the most lethal in all of the world and has been linked with contributing to illness rather than to promoting health. Peoples who rely on real, unrefined plant foods to nourish them have been shown to have much less cancer in general than those who rely on the typical American diet.

IN SEARCH OF ENERGY AND CARBOHYDRATES

The first need of the body, after water, is energy. No one would doubt that we need energy to survive. During treatment, soon after treatment ends, and later when you feel well enough to consider yourself recovered and normal, the primary need of the body is *energy*. *"What kinds of foods will help us have more energy?"* is one of the most commonly asked questions. But often during recovery from cancer, because of the aftereffects of treatment, you may have a *run down* digestive system and a limited desire to eat. You may feel that you cannot even look at foods, or you may be experiencing some nausea or other digestive upsets just when, more than ever, you have a desperate need for energy. This energy has to come from that food you are rejecting.

No matter how inactive or active a person is—from you who are now recovering from your cancer to the elite marathon runner who uses hundreds of calories in just a few hours—that person needs energy to be alive. Even when asleep, the body uses energy to perform such basic tasks as keeping warm, keeping the heart pumping blood, and keeping the lungs inhaling and exhaling air. Unfortunately, many of us associate calories with getting fat, not getting better. For now, forget any concerns or fears you may have about calories in foods.

The easiest to digest calories and the ones that give us energy soon after eating are the carbohydrates. A loaf of whole grain bread was the preferred source of energy of the Roman armies at the peak of the Roman Empire. It gave them plenty of good digestible carbohydrates, together with protein and fiber.

If we eat enough carbohydrates each day—about 400 calories' worth—the body's biochemical machinery works better than if we rely only on protein or fat for energy. Over an entire day, four hundred calories add up fast. For example, it takes only one cup of cooked whole wheat pasta or brown rice, two servings of fresh fruits and vegetables, and a quarter cup of sun-dried raisins to give you about 400 calories—or in sippable terms, a drink made with one cup lowfat yogurt and one cup nectar will give you close to that much.

With the exception of milk, carbohydrates come from plants. Milk contains a sugar that, as you would expect, is called milk sugar (to the chemist, this sugar is known as lactose). The best sources of carbohydrates are found in grains, fresh and dried fruits, dry beans, peas, lentils, and starchy vegetables like potatoes, carrots, and other root vegetables. These are the foods that give you, together with the energy from carbohydrates, a powerhouse of healing and protective compounds in each bite; this is in contrast to white sugar and foods made with white flour, which give you mostly just calories, not to mention other added artificial ingredients that your already stressed body must handle. Nuts and oily seeds such as sesame and sunflower contain some carbohydrates, but they also contain larger amounts of fat and protein. You won't find carbohydrates in animal foods like meat, poultry, cheese, butter, cream cheese, or lard, or in vegetable oils.

In a Nutshell
While undergoing treatment and in the early days after treatment ends, forget your fears about calories. The secret now is to eat enough easily digestible food for energy, while trying to get all the health-enhancing and protective factors possible.

In the early stages of recovery, it may be useful to add properly formulated, super-easy-to-digest, complete liquid or powder supplements to your diet (see page 20). Our recipes for "Super Sippables" (page 83) show you some combinations of liquid foods that are high in energy, are easy to digest, and which are powerhouses of healing and protective compounds.

THE BUILDING AND HEALING POWER OF PROTEINS

Proteins play a crucial role in the healing process. While protein gives us energy—it can be broken down by the body into sugars or fats if needed—the key functions of proteins are to build and rebuild the body, help it to perform vital, life-sustaining functions, and protect us from illness. To many people the word protein means foods like beef, pork, lamb, chicken, or cheese. While these are good reliable protein sources, many animal foods are high in saturated fat, the kind of fat you want to keep low because it has been linked to various chronic diseases.

Too often people think that we must eat animal foods like meat to get enough of the right kind of protein. But traditional wisdom and history tells us differently. Many civilizations have thrived on eating patterns with little or no meat. Today, groups that eat very little or no animal foods tend to be healthier than those who rely on it as their staple food. Instead of animal foods, these peoples get their protein from plants. Of special interest to the cancer survivor, and to help prevent future recurrence, is the fact that some types of cancer are higher in populations that consume large amounts of animal foods, especially meat. In a study of a Seventh Day Adventist population in California, regular meat eaters had more pancreatic cancer than non-meat eaters.

The highest quality protein in the plant world is found in cooked dry beans, lentils, whole grains, and in nuts. It is not

In a Nutshell
When using grains, cereals, and flours, always choose the unrefined, whole grain products.

difficult to get all the protein you need from these plant foods. When your appetite is poor, your system stressed by treatments, and you want soft, easy-to-chew, and digestible foods that the body finds easy to handle, protein foods such as tofu from soybeans—one of the great plant proteins—and nonfat or lowfat dairy foods like milk, cottage or ricotta cheese, and yogurt, are all excellent sources.

But what about eggs? Egg proteins are at the top of every list of good body building proteins. It is one of the most easily digested and best utilized proteins for building and rebuilding body tissues. The white of the egg is just about pure protein, while the yolk, as we all know, contains enough cholesterol to worry many people. While under treatment or in the early stages of recovery, the goodness of the egg protein must outweigh the cholesterol concerns, unless your physician or health professional has advised you to limit your cholesterol intake. If you have been told to avoid whole eggs, remember that you can use the white of the egg, totally cholesterol-free. Indeed, a piece of whole grain toast topped with an egg may be just the perfect thing to help you get started in the morning or to keep you going on days when you aren't feeling well. However, when things are going well and you are well on your way to recovery, getting most of your protein from plants should be your first choice.

FATS: HARMFUL OR BENEFICIAL?

Just about every day you read about lowfat foods, a new oil-free salad dressing, an artificial fat substitute. Does this mean that fat is some kind of evil entity placed by nature into so many of our *natural* foods to hurt us? The answer is no; there are many good fats. However, since fats are such a concentrated food, it makes sense to eat them only in moderation.

The secret to eating fats in health and cancer prevention is simple:

1. The *good and safe fats* are found in nuts and seeds—like almonds, walnuts, hazelnuts, sesame and sunflower seeds, their oils and "butters," avocados, and extra virgin olive oil or unrefined sesame oil. Good fats are also present in the germ of grains and in soy products like tofu.

2. Avoid excesses of saturated fats, usually animal fats, with the exception of fish. Eat only small amounts of animal products, like beef, pork, lamb, whole milk and milk products, butter, cream cheese, lard, and bacon fat. It's fairly clear that a diet high in saturated fat increases at least the risk for colorectal cancer.

3. Use plant oils in moderation, but don't be afraid of natural plant oils as they are mostly unsaturated, with the exception of coconut and certain kinds of palm oils.

4. Avoid artificially prepared fats (also called trans fats or trans fatty acids) like hydrogenated fats in shortening, some margarines, and many commercial baked goods and snack foods. Artificially prepared fats have some of the same properties as saturated fats, although their role in cancer is unclear at this time.

Unrefined oils, like extra virgin olive oil and that from nuts and oily seeds such as sesame and wheat germ, are among the good fats that contain powerful, natural, disease-fighting antioxidants. More about antioxidants later. For a cancer patient, these kinds of fats are probably the safest, as shown by a recent Greek study, where women consuming olive oil had a very low occurrence of breast cancer.

The healthiest kinds of oils to buy are those that have been processed only by cold pressing: These are minimally processed and ultimately retain the maximum amount of their naturally occurring health-protecting substances. You may, however, have to go to a health food store or a market that sells whole foods to find cold pressed oils.

While under treatment you may not feel like eating "fat," as fat is sometimes not as easy to handle with a digestive system under the stress of certain chemotherapies. But later, after your digestive system is well again, a moderate amount of fat in the diet does seem to be beneficial to total health, and in fact, the body must have a very small amount of fat to work properly—probably just a few teaspoons each day. Just remember that extremes—too little or too much of anything—are never desirable.

VITAMINS AND MINERALS

Many of the healing and protective components, vitamins and minerals, of plants are present in very small amounts. They do not supply energy like carbohydrates or fats, or building blocks for tissues and cells like proteins. For a long time we have known about the significance of vitamins and minerals—that they are essential to health and life itself; that they don't give us energy; and that some are needed to turn proteins, carbohydrates, and fats into energy. But we need to focus on four functions vital to recovery for the cancer survivor.

First of all, B vitamins, such as thiamin, riboflavin, and niacin, are key factors in the production of energy from carbohydrates and fats.

Secondly, B vitamins help the digestive system to work properly. Two good examples are thiamin and niacin: Thiamin is known to stimulate appetite and niacin deficiency is known to cause diarrhea. There is no doubt that without enough of these B vitamins, the digestive system does not function properly.

Thirdly, some B vitamins like folate (folic acid) and B_{12} are critical for blood cell production, often a common problem during treatment.

Finally, during treatment and later when totally recovered, some vitamins like vitamin C, beta-carotene (a plant source of vitamin A), and vitamin E and its related compounds (called tocopherols) are powerful "protectors" against chronic diseases like cancer. They are not magic wands that can assure us of permanent health—life processes always depend on a wide array of factors—but they are key protective substances. *A key property they share is that they are all powerful antioxidants.*

Whole grains and cooked dry beans are high in B vitamins; berries, oranges and other citrus fruits, kiwis, and sweet peppers are high in vitamin C; yellow and orange fleshed and dark green leafy vegetables give us carotenes (which include beta-carotene as well as other members of the large carotene family); and nuts are especially good sources of vitamin E and related antioxidants. Whole grains and wheat germ oil also supply vitamin E (notice how whole grains are a storehouse of so many different good things). It's vital to remember, too, that these B vitamins and vitamin C are *water soluble* and that the body loses them very rapidly, more so than vitamin E or carotenes, which are insoluble in water and are stored in the body. This means that we should eat abundantly, every single day, of the foods that supply water soluble vitamins. However, even though beta-carotene and vitamin E are lost less from the body, we should still eat, on a rather frequent basis, abundantly of foods that provide these important nutrients.

The need for vitamins and minerals cannot be overemphasized—but equally important is to obtain them from unrefined, minimally processed foods. However, a good supplement supplying the Recommended Dietary Allowances for vitamins and minerals can help. Some vitamins like A and D should never be taken in excess of the recommended intakes. Vitamin E, beta-carotene, and vitamin C may be taken in moderately larger amounts. But never use a supplement in place of a good diet, use it in addition to a good diet! You may be missing out on so much without even knowing it!

In a Nutshell

Antioxidants prevent the body from damage by stifling or fending off, the out of control action of unstable compounds (called free radicals).

THE MAGIC OF FIBER AND PHYTOCHEMICALS

There was a time when it seemed as though we knew all we needed to know about nutrition and health. But, you may ask, what about all those compounds in foods, literally hundreds of them, that are neither vitamins, minerals, proteins, fats, or digestible carbohydrates? Did we think they were just colors or flavors or structural parts of the plant, important to the plant but not valuable to us? In the past 20 or 30 years, a treasure chest of beneficial compounds in plants has emerged as crucial in cancer prevention.

A major development in the history of this *new* nutrition took place in the late 1960s and early 1970s when *fiber* from plants was found to be important for good health and helpful to lowering risk for diseases, such as cancer. It's important to think about that since we eat a lot of fiber-depleted foods, such as refined grains (like white rice and pastas) and white flour baked products (like cakes, cookies, and pastries). Less than 10 percent of us eat anywhere near the amount of fruits and vegetables each day that we should. A meal of meat, mashed potatoes, and green beans with a French roll and apple pie is a typical fiber-deprived meal that too many people eat on a day-to-day basis.

Fiber is found only in plants. There are two basic types: insoluble and soluble. To get a good balance between them, each of which has its own health benefits, you do not have to be an expert or even read labels: Simply be sure to include in your diet plenty of whole grains, cooked dry beans, lentils and peas, nuts and seeds, and fresh or dried fruits and vegetables. In addition, high fiber foods are nature's storehouse for other healthful substances. For example, grapes and sun-dried raisins contain not only a good balance of fibers, but tartaric acid, a phytochemical that we have recently studied in our research center that helps proper bowel function, which is sometimes a difficulty experienced by cancer patients. Most foods contain both kinds of fiber, but in different proportions—unless the food has been processed or refined. Whole wheat flour literally becomes fiber depleted and provides little health benefit to the digestive tract when it is made into white flour. Choosing minimally processed plant foods will help assure you of getting lots of good fibers.

More recently, during the eighties, the era of *phytochemicals* was born, and it has reached explosive proportions in the early nineties. Today phytochemicals are the focus of extensive research all over the world. There are literally hundreds, maybe even thousands, of these substances found plentifully in plants. Many phytochemicals have health-promoting and disease-preventing properties, and many have been linked with anti-cancer action, such as slowing down cancer development by delaying tumor growth and possibly reversing precancerous tumors before they become malignant. Some have been linked to heart disease prevention. Other phytochemicals have been shown to boost the immune system and protect cells from attack by cancer-causing compounds by acting as antioxidants. Some of the key phytochemicals in foods are the:

Carotenoids, which include hundreds of related substances and give the characteristic colors to fruits and vegetables, such as *beta-carotene* found in dark green and yellow- or orange-fleshed vegetables; *lycopene,* found in tomatoes; and *lutein,* found in spinach and other green leaves. They have been shown to help the body combat cancer and its progression.

Allylic sulfides, which are especially abundant in garlic and other vegetables of the onion family. Many studies have shown that these phytochemicals have: beneficial interactions with the immune system, tumor-fighting action, blood coagulation and heart disease control, and bacteria-killing properties.

Phenolic compounds, which include many hundreds of substances, like the currently popular *flavonoids.* These have been found to be powerful antioxidants and anti-tumor agents. They are present in many fruits, vegetables, cooked dry beans, and unrefined whole grains. Red wine, dark beer, and green and black tea also contain phenolic compounds.

Phytoestrogens, which are found in soybean products like tofu. These deserve to be highlighted for the cancer survivor since they have been found to be important cancer-protective agents.

Plant sterols, which have been studied since the 1950s but were then forgotten. Plant sterols are found in oils, nuts and seeds, whole grains, and cooked dry beans. Although renewed interest in their benefits has emerged only in recent years, they seem to protect against cancer as well as to help lower blood cholesterol.

Phytates, usually found together with fiber in grains, beans, and vegetables. These have been shown in animals to protect against some chemically-induced cancers.

This is only a partial list—there are so many protective compounds that in recent years whole books have been written about phytochemicals—but what's really critical to remember is that we have just begun to uncover this treasure of precious plant compounds that show health-enhancing properties, and that only in wholesome, unrefined foods—especially fruits, vegetables, grains, and legumes—can we be sure to find them. When in a few years you read that a new compound "X" has been found in some fruit, nut, oily seed, vegetable, whole grain, or bean, you'll be able to say to yourself: "I have been eating that food all along, much before science would tell me it was healthy!" This is a very important point, if you put it in a historical perspective. For example, many Asian peoples have eaten soybean products like tofu for centuries, and just recently we have discovered that the phytoestrogens in soybeans may protect against breast cancer!

Unfortunately, many common foods in the typical American diet have literally processed out much of the phytochemicals nature had put in, along with vitamins, minerals, and good fibers. One of the facts that reminds us that we should eat an abundance of unrefined foods is the almost certain presence of an array of as yet unidentified substances, which may turn out to be necessary for healing and protection!

WATER, THE OVERLOOKED NUTRIENT

We all take water for granted, so its tremendous role in health is often overlooked. Think of your body as being mostly water, over 60 percent. Consider that some scientists think of aging as a process of dehydration. Consider that the first requirement of an endurance athlete like a long distance runner or bicyclist is water—dehydration is one of the first causes of fatigue.

Plain, good water, fresh juices, teas—herbal or otherwise—should be consumed as a regular part of our daily routine. Choose the source of fluid you like, but make it a key part of your diet. Green tea appears to be rich in phenols that have tumor-protective properties, but remember that it also contains caffeine, a stimulant. Coffee should be consumed with more caution: The scientific community does not agree as to whether large consumption of coffee may favor the development of some cancers, but some correlation was found in the same Seventh Day Adventist study we mentioned earlier. The cancer survivor should be extra cautious, so choose tea over coffee, or limit your coffee consumption to an occasional treat.

In a Nutshell

Whole, unrefined plant foods are carriers of much protection. Make them the foundation of your diet at any time and even more so during periods of stress. Let these foods supply most of your protein, energy, fat, vitamins, minerals, fibers, and superprotective phytochemicals.

Water has no energy but is most essential to life. Remember the vital role of fluid intake and drink abundantly every day.

Chapter 2

THE KEY FOODS FOR RESTORING AND MAINTAINING HEALTH

YOU ARE NOW READY TO CHOOSE THE FOODS THAT should be your first choices during treatment and after recovery. Foods that are rich in health-giving components and that have no *negatives* are the best choices at all times. Remember that the greatest potential for restoring your body's health and replenishing your body's stores comes from a diet that is based on foods from plants.

THE ART OF EATING WELL

Eating properly is an art. It's an art that will empower you to make the best choices and to optimize the healing and recovery processes, especially when you're not feeling well and eating is an unpleasant chore. The optimal food plan during treatment and recovery is far from being unconventional. It is a way of eating that is purely and simply natural.

There are two sides when it comes to choosing the best possible foods for the recovery and prevention of future cancers. On one side you need to make superprotective and building foods the cornerstones of your meals; on the other side you need to avoid, as much as possible, foods that may be low in protective factors or that have possible negative effects—effects that a healthy body may overcome but that the cancer survivor needs to avoid as much as possible.

CHOOSING THE BEST NOURISHING AND PROTECTING FOODS

In a Nutshell

The cutting edge of research shows that a diet based primarily on whole, minimally processed plant foods is the best choice.

You have probably noticed that the majority of the foods that are optimal for eating during cancer treatment and recovery come from the earth. These foods also come equipped with millennia of human experience, and this experience has shown us that, not only are these foods not harmful, but that they have healthful advantages. Most of us eat some of these precious gems from the earth once in a while, but they are not the foundation of our meals. The difference for the cancer survivor is that they must become the central ingredients in eating, instead of just a pretty garnish.

Your individual tolerances for certain foods may limit what choices you will be able to make, but don't despair and don't forget about them. Remind yourself that something you couldn't tolerate, chew, or swallow one week, or even one day, may be acceptable or appealing the next day or next week. Allow yourself to be open and flexible about swings in appetite and food preferences at this time. You owe it to yourself.

Optimal foods are those that are at the top of the list in terms of nutrient content. Many are easy to prepare, and can be tolerated well and easily handled even if you have a sensitive stomach or problems chewing and swallowing. They also have the added bonus of being money saving when they take the place of many expensive animal and nutrient-depleted, modern designer foods. Choose your foods as you would choose a precious gem from the earth.

Because of the added demands on your body and the potential aftereffects of treatment during recovery, a few foods from the animal kingdom harmonize well with plant foods to enhance your health and eating enjoyment. These healthy additions are *nonfat and lowfat milk and yogurt, part skim ricotta cheese and cottage cheese,* and very digestible, edible, and easy-to-prepare eggs. More than anyone else, though, the cancer survivor has to overcome the "meat as a main dish" mentality, which is all too prevalent in today's American lifestyle. You can get all the nutrition you need, along with the bonus pack of phytochemicals, from plant foods with some milk and egg proteins.

Never forget that for millennia our ancestors have combined pasta or rice with vegetables and beans, tofu with rice, and beans with corn and bread. Many great civilizations were founded and still thrive on these staple foods.

THE KEY NOURISHING AND PROTECTING GEMS

Let's find the great foods that belong to the optimal diet. They are listed in the table that follows ("Gems for the Optimal Diet"). You'll find a large number of luscious foods that range from the delicate and light whole grain of millet to hearty legumes. Foods with an asterisk after their name are also good sources of protein. In Chapter 4 you'll find out ways to make these foods meet special situations, such as the times when the food has to be very easy to digest.

There are no refined sugars, refined flours or grains, hydrogenated or high saturated fat foods in this list. Remember that candies, pastries, and cakes are often made with these ingredients. Sometimes too much salt or too many chemicals are added that your body, already stressed by the treatment, must work to handle them. These kinds of foods should not be part of your regular eating pattern. Whole grain cakes and other desserts made with vegetable oils and unrefined sugar and eggs or egg whites can be highly nutritious: If you can find or are willing to prepare this kind of cake or pastry, keep them handy for extra special treats.

THE GREEN-ORANGE LAW, KEY TO THE SELECTION OF FRUITS AND VEGETABLES

One simple and all-important principle that can be used when choosing vegetables and fruits, is what we call the *green-orange law*, which we introduced in one of our recent books (*Eat Your Way to Better Health*).

If, in the same group of vegetables, one is white and another has lots of green or orange or other dark colors, pick the dark-colored one! For example, in the cabbage family, the green or dark-colored broccoli and some purple-green cauliflowers are richer in nutrients than white cauliflower. Similarly, carrots, which are orange in color, have an abundance of carotenes compared to white root, underground vegetables like potatoes.

When you apply this *green-orange law*, be sure to base your choices on the color of the pulp of the vegetable or fruit, not on the color of its skin or rind. There are some great choices that are mild and tender—like winter squashes in their many varieties, carrots, orange pulp sweet potatoes, spinach, and dark green or red lettuces. Winter squashes, carrots, and sweet potatoes are especially easy to make creamy smooth so that they are easier to swallow and digest.

THE ROLES OF SUPPLEMENTS AND PREPARED LIQUID DIETS

To insure a reasonable intake of vitamins and minerals, the cancer survivor can find comfort in a proper nutrient supplement or prepared liquid or powder meal replacement. Ask your health

Gems for the Optimal Diet

Grains	Fruits	Vegetables	Legumes
Amaranth*	Apples	Artichokes	Cooked dry beans*
Barley (best: hulled)*	Apricots	Asparagus	Lentils*
Brown Rice*	Avocados	Beets	Nuts and seeds and
Buckwheat*	Bananas	Broccoli, Brussels	their butters*
Bulgur or cracked	Berries (blueberries,	sprouts, cauliflower,	Soy milk*
wheat*	strawberries, etc.)	kohlrabi	Split Peas
Couscous (best: whole	Cantaloupe and other	Cabbage	Tempeh*
wheat)*	melons	Carrots	Tofu*
Millet*	Cherries	Corn	
Pasta and noodles (best:	Citrus fruit	Celery	
whole wheat)*	Dates	Dark green salad and	
Quinoa*	Figs	leafy greens	
Rice (best: brown)*	Grapes	(romaine, red leaf,	
Stone ground polenta or	Kiwifruit and other	spinach, chard, kale,	
cornmeal*	exotic fruits	collards, etc.)	
Wheat germ*	Mangos	Eggplant	
Whole grain breads and	Nectarines	Fennel (anise)	
cereals* with or with-	Nectars, natural juices	Fresh green beans	
out nuts or seeds	Papayas	Garlic	
Whole wheat couscous*	Peaches	Mushrooms	
Wild rice*	Pears	Onions (yellow, white,	
	Persimmons	red, and green, leeks)	
	Plums	Parsley	
	Prunes	Parsnips, turnips, and	
	Pumpkins	rutabagas	
	Sun-dried raisins and	Peas, fresh green	
	other dried fruits	Peppers, red or green	
	Tomatoes	Potatoes (all kinds)	
		Purslane	
		Sprouts	
		Summer squash (zuc-	
		chini, etc.)	
		Sweet potatoes, yams	
		Vegetable juices	
		Winter squashes	
		(banana, butternut,	
		Danish, kabocha, etc.)	

*Good source of protein.

Gems for the Optimal Diet (*continued*)

Good Fats	Herbs and Spices	Animal Foods	Sweeteners
Almond oil	Basil	Cottage cheese* (best: nonfat or very low-fat)	Brown or other unrefined sugars
Avocado oil	Bay leaves		Honey
Avocados	Chamomile		Maple syrup (100% pure—not artificially flavored)
Extra virgin olive oil	Dill	Egg whites or whole eggs*	
Hazelnut oil	Fennel		
Nut butters (almond and others)	Ginger	Kefir*	Molasses
Seed butters (tahini and others)	Chile peppers	Milk* (best: nonfat or lowfat 1%)	
	Lavender		
Sesame oil	Lemongrass	Yogurt* (best: without gelatin or thickeners)	
Wheat germ oil	Marjoram		
	Nasturtium		
	Oregano		
	Peppermint (and other mints)		
	Rosemary		
	Sage		
	Savory		
	Sorrel		
	Tarragon		
	Thyme		

*Good source of protein.

professional about the supplement formula you choose, to be sure it is a good choice.

There are three types of supplements to consider:

1. A basic, all around supplement that supplies the Recommended Dietary Intakes (RDIs are the recommended amounts of nutrients listed on supplement labels) of all the known essential vitamins and minerals. This kind of supplement is intended to reassure us that if we do not balance our diet properly and/or if our system is not well and our digestion poor, that we take in the required amount of all essential vitamins and

minerals every day. This can be especially important for a body under stress or one that has recently undergone a stressful event.

2. Supplements that contain protective vitamins in amounts larger than the RDI. Here you need to be careful: Never supplement vitamins A, D, and K beyond the RDI unless recommended by a health professional. They are water insoluble and are stored in your body; and taking too much can create toxic levels in your blood. Supplementing in reasonable excesses beyond RDIs with antioxidant vitamins, E, C, and beta-carotene has been shown to be relatively safe. B vitamins are also safe in moderate excesses, and may help your appetite in the early stages of recovery.

3. Liquid meals. There are some excellent prepared *liquid meals* that supply total basic nutrition for those who have problems consuming solid food. Look for a reliable manufacturer and be sure the label states that it supplies complete nutrition. Except when very sick and unable to eat anything else, liquid meals should not be used to replace every meal in a day: Make one or two meals a liquid meal and plan your other meals around the *Supereasy* recipes in this book (page 41). Or use liquid meals to give you more calories as a supplement to your regular whole food meals.

WHAT KINDS OF FOODS SHOULD YOU EAT LESS OFTEN?

Some commercially prepared *designer* foods are so manipulated that what may have been a storehouse of all the possible goodness of the earth may now just be a depleted convenience food in a pretty package. As the first ingredient on a label is the one present in the largest amount (by law), avoid prepared or designer foods that list first a refined sugar or wheat flour, or enriched wheat flour (if it had been made with the whole grain, the words *whole wheat flour* would have appeared). When the first ingredient is a refined food like sugar or white flour, it means that you're largely getting a nutrient-depleted product—that is, many vitamins, minerals, protective compounds, and fiber were removed. If you choose prepared foods, choose the ones that list only whole, unrefined ingredients on the label, such as a bread made with whole wheat flour, dried fruits, honey, and nuts.

In other foods, some substances that may potentially harm or aggravate a condition may be present due to the way they were prepared. In deep fat frying, when fats are heated at high temperatures, chemical changes take place that alter the structure of the fat molecule in undesirable ways. These potentially toxic substances are called *trans fatty acids*. Some scientists are finding that these trans fatty acids may contribute to the development of chronic disease. In charbroiling, a particularly harmful chemical is formed when animal fats drip onto hot charcoal during the broiling of meats: The fat decomposes and forms compounds that are considered cancer-producing (these compounds are called polycyclic aromatic hydrocarbons). Some of these compounds are then adsorbed by the charbroiling foods and the result is a food that is probably best avoided. You may be more sensitive to compounds that may be tolerated by other people, and fried or broiled meats may be risky. The best ways to prepare your food are to microwave, boil, stew, or bake them. When you do use fat, cook with the good fats (like olive oil) over low to moderate heat.

Some scientists have also found a possible connection between foods that have high amounts of salt, nitrates, and nitrites in them and certain cancers. Typically, these substances are found in processed meats and salty and pickled foods. Studies have shown that the Japanese, who eat a lot of dried salted fish and pickled vegetables, have a much higher incidence of stomach cancer than peoples in other cultures. And as toxic substances may develop in moldy food, be sure to discard any foods that have any trace of mold.

A WORD ABOUT COMFORT FOODS

Foods that help us feel better when we think about them are often called *comfort foods*. These are the foods that many people think of first when they are not feeling well. They are usually good sources of calories, but often that's all they give us, as they are nutrient-depleted foods like cakes and cookies. If while under treatment you occasionally crave some foods made with these refined ingredients, remember that the need for energy should temporarily override other considerations. Go ahead and eat that cake or candy, as long as you remember that it should only be an *emergency* food. Switch to whole grains or other whole, unrefined food as soon as you can.

DR. POTTER ON FRUITS AND VEGETABLES

by John D. Potter, MD, PhD, Head, Cancer Prevention Research Program Fred Hutchinson Cancer Research Center, Seattle, Washington

Over the past decade, a substantial number of studies have examined the effect of plant food consumption on health and disease. The finding that high intakes of vegetables and fruit are protective against many human cancers is better supported by the scientific literature than almost all other dietary hypotheses about cancer.

Over 200 studies have been conducted in many different parts of the world to investigate the role of vegetables and fruit in altering the risk of cancer in different organs of the body. The evidence strongly suggests that it is not the consumption of one or two varieties of vegetables and fruit that confer benefit, but rather that intake of many different kinds of plant foods is higher in those at lower risk of cancer. The fact that individuals who consume higher intakes of vegetables also have other healthy habits, such as a lower likelihood of smoking, does not account for all of the differences seen.

It's clear that many people do not eat enough vegetables and fruit. For any community or even nation, some specific incentives for the production of more vegetables and fruit would allow the changes at the individual level to be made more easily and, ultimately, may prove to be a useful investment in lowering the burden of chronic disease.

Chapter 3

HERBS, SPICES, TEAS, AND THE MAGIC OF CLUSTERING

FOR CENTURIES PEOPLE OF EVERY CONTINENT HAVE used herbs, spices, and teas to flavor foods and make beverages. While we all know that kitchen herbs can turn a simple dish into a gourmet meal, we forget that many kitchen herbs and spices were at one time considered to have beneficial and medicinal properties. Today, scientists have confirmed that many of them contain potent compounds with antioxidant and cancer-protective properties. Nature in her wisdom gave enticing aroma to these plants so that humans would want to use them to make beverages or to flavor bland foods like rice.

Logically, the presence in a dish of a touch of a protective herb or spice—be it rosemary or allspice—is not going to do much to add either flavor or biological protection. But herbs and spices can add to a healthful, protective meal if you use them frequently and use a sufficient amount, such as a sprig of rosemary fresh from the garden—not just a small pinch. This is the first key concept that applies not only to herbs but to all other components of our meals.

The second key concept to designing *a protective meal* is that we must consider the beneficial action of an herb (or any other food) not in isolation but *as one of many contributors to the total sum of beneficial nutrients and phytochemicals in that meal.* A good way to think about the way good (or bad!) things add up in a person's diet is to think of how money works: A large amount of money is nothing more than the sum of single dollars. A good technique for visualizing how herbs, spices, teas, and all other foods work together is *clustering.* More on clustering later in this chapter.

STAR HERBS AND SPICES—STOREHOUSES OF FLAVOR AND PROTECTION

Many Japanese researchers, inspired by the long Asian tradition of respect for herbal medicine, have led the way in the search for protective compounds in herbs and spices. Here are just a few common herbs and spices that are high in antioxidants.

Rosemary, sage, thyme, oregano, marjoram, and basil
Ginger, turmeric, and cardamom
Mace and its inner part nutmeg
Bay leaves and cinnamon
Allspice and cloves
Cumin and fennel seeds

Laboratory studies have shown that many of the compounds in these herbs, in sufficient quantities, have potent inhibitory effects on cancer cells. Early botanists knew it when they gave Latin names to some herbs—which is another reflection of the ancient wisdom we often tend to downplay in our modern, highly technological world. Yes, our ancestors knew more about health than most of us give them credit for.

OUR ANCESTORS KNEW

Much can be learned by studying what our ancestors did in their wisdom, much before modern chemistry. Here is a good example: When centuries ago early botanists began to give Latin names to plants, the term *officinalis* was often given to plants that were considered to have beneficial or medicinal properties. The term comes from *officina* (or other related Latin terms), which is an ancient drug shop, an herb store, or a pharmacy where medicinal herbs were sold. The two common herbs that include *officinalis* in their Latin name are sage, *Salvia officinalis,* and rosemary, *Rosmarinus officinalis.* An unfounded belief of early medicine? Not at all: We know today that these two herbs contain potent antioxidants with exotic names like carnositic acid, carnosol, and ursolic acid. But these two and many other herbs have more than just antioxidant properties. Sage was and is still used as a tea for inflammation of the mouth and throat and for digestive complaints. Similarly, rosemary is often recommended for digestive upsets, flatulence, and to stimulate appetite and stomach secretions. Rosemary is such a good antioxidant that it has been used in foods as a natural preservative of meats and fats for years. Entire books have been written about all the herbs in common use; rosemary and sage are used here just as examples of the potential protective properties of herbs. As soon as you feel well enough to tolerate their flavors, use them!

And remember: Fresh herbs usually have a higher content of these compounds than dry ones. If you grow herbs in your garden, use them often, use them fresh, use enough; and if you dry them, do it gently.

CHILE PEPPERS

This is a spice you may choose to use when feeling normal. There are many varieties of chile peppers, and originating in South

America, they have conquered the world. In many people's minds they are associated more with Middle Eastern or Indian cooking than with their origin in Peru and the ancient Incas. They range from quite mild to extremely hot and the amount used varies accordingly. The key substance that makes chile peppers popular is *capsaicin,* which is a biologically active substance often used in ointments as a pain killer. In moderation, chile peppers bring life to food and help digestion. But if your digestive tract is sensitive, you may prefer to avoid hot chile peppers in the early days of treatment and recovery.

GINGER

Ginger grows wild in the tropical forests of Southeast Asia and is one of the foundations of Indian cookery and an essential part of Asian spice mixtures. It is also an essential ingredient of curry. Our ancestors recognized the antiseptic power of ginger by using it as an antidote for the plague that besieged Europe in the Middle Ages. Ancient Chinese sailors used ginger to prevent scurvy, long before the English used limes in the eighteenth century. In 1993, researchers at the City University of Osaka in Japan found not one, but 21 compounds in ginger—some of them, as you would expect, are called gingerols—with various antioxidant powers. And some of these ginger compounds were found to be more powerful antioxidants than vitamin E. The antimicrobial and antioxidant properties of ginger were also recognized in the past, in another way: Ginger was known to be a good natural food preservative.

Recently ginger has been found to be beneficial for motion sickness and nausea. A delicious, soothing, and healthful tea can be made with either fresh or dry ginger. A note of caution: Ginger is a good all-around herb for the cancer survivor *when not on chemotherapy.* During chemotherapy it may not be desirable, as ginger acts as an anticoagulant. You should check with your doctor before using it in large amounts, notwithstanding its stomach-calming benefits.

CHINESE AND INDIAN TEAS

You may not consider Chinese or Indian teas as herbs, but thousands of years ago ancient peoples discovered that leaves other than those we now call kitchen herbs, leaves like tea, also had healthful properties. One of these is the common Chinese or Indian tea leaf (*Camelia sinensis*). The leaves of the tea plant were considered, in the wisdom of ancient Chinese people, almost sacred, and they were believed to possess great healing powers.

Today we know that tea leaves are a rich source of antioxidants. All Chinese and Indian teas, especially green and the more rare *white* teas, are a rich source of a group of antioxidants called polyphenols. In several Japanese studies (the Japanese consume large amounts of tea) these compounds have been found to have cancer-preventing properties. Be aware, though, that there is caffeine and some related compounds in tea, so avoid these types of tea when you want to rest or if you are caffeine sensitive. And even though we have said this before, let's remember that each one of these protective foods should be looked at as a part of the entire picture of our daily routine, and not as magic substances in isolation.

THE SECRETS OF CLUSTERING

Clusters are a great visual way to help us recognize how the sum of small amounts of protective factors found in foods—that in isolation may not be sufficient to do us much good—become meaningful when we add together all the foods that we eat in a day. *Clustering* makes us aware of how this works. The truth of clustering is often overlooked and we may say: ". . . a little rosemary or sage is not going to make any difference." Probably true, if your only phytochemicals came from these herbs. But combine them with vitamin E, fiber and phytates from whole grains, carotenes from green leaves, polyphenols from tea, vitamin C

In a Nutshell
While the small amount of herbs added to a dish or in a cup of tea may supply little in the way of protective factors, it is the sum of all the factors in a meal that counts. We must get away from looking at each food in isolation: We need to look at an entire day of food and beverage consumption as a whole.

from lemon juice, and many other compounds from plant foods, and the picture becomes impressive. *Never forget that each little bite of food counts.*

The first figure that follows is an example of the clustering of good foods (see Figure 3.1). It's followed by a figure with blank ovals that you can photocopy and use to see how your various foods, herbs, and beverages work in your chosen diet (see Figure 3.2). Make each oval count. The third figure helps you visualize what happens when many of these ovals are filled with refined, low protective foods (see Figure 3.3). Try it! The final results—and your meals—will be quite different.

Figure 3.1 *A Cluster of Superfoods*

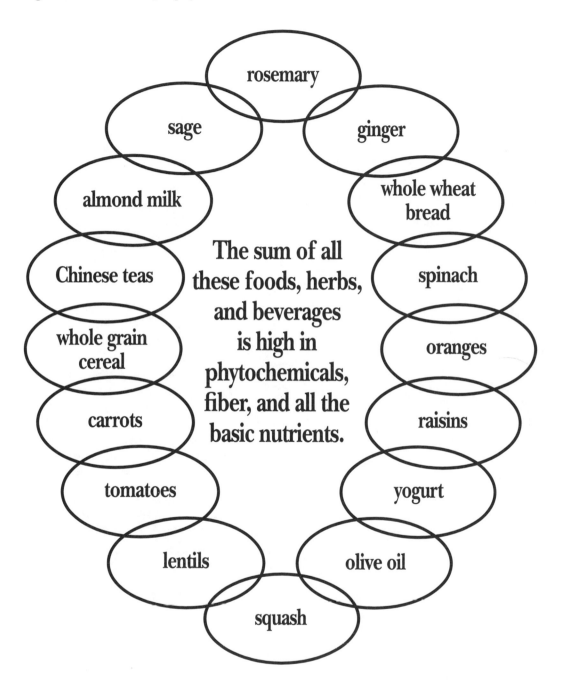

rosemary

sage

ginger

almond milk

whole wheat bread

Chinese teas

spinach

The sum of all these foods, herbs, and beverages is high in phytochemicals, fiber, and all the basic nutrients.

whole grain cereal

oranges

carrots

raisins

tomatoes

yogurt

lentils

olive oil

squash

Figure 3.2   *Test Your Diet*

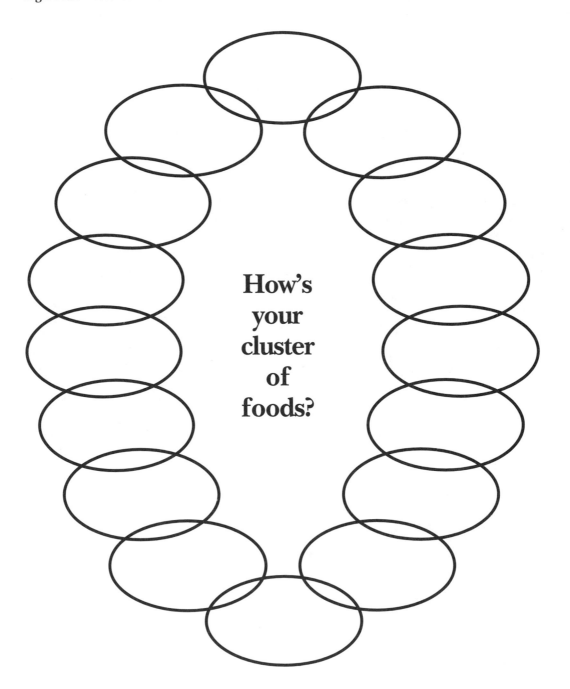

How's
your
cluster
of
foods?

Figure 3.3   *A Cluster of Mixed Foods*

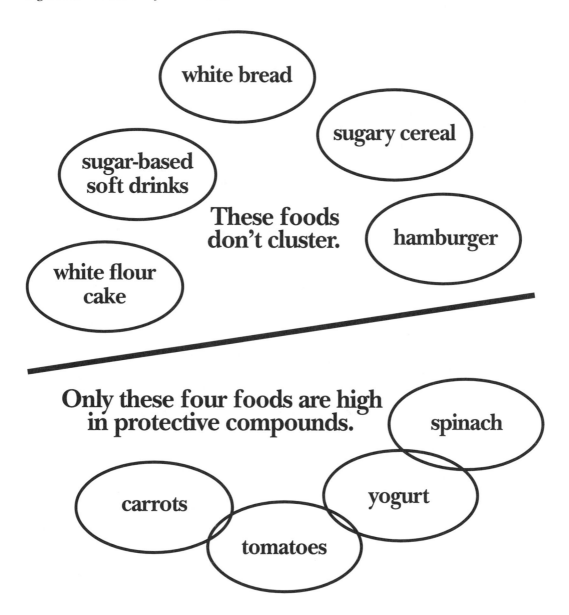

Chapter 4

PUTTING IT ALL TOGETHER: THE CANCER SURVIVOR'S PYRAMID

MANY *FOOD PYRAMIDS* HAVE BEEN DESIGNED SINCE THE early 1970s to help people choose the best possible diet. There is a United States Department of Agriculture (USDA) *Food Guide Pyramid,* a Mediterranean and an Asian pyramid, Norwegian and Swedish pyramids, and many others. In addition, there is our own Superpyramid. The Cancer Survivor's Pyramid, however, is a very special one in particular. *This pyramid is unique and a departure from all other pyramids.* It is designed to show you how the optimum foods we have been talking about fit in with the various special needs of the cancer survivor.

THE SUPERPYRAMID

The Superpyramid (from Gene Spiller's *Eat Your Way to Better Health*) is an example of a food pyramid that can be useful to

Figure 4.1   The Superpyramid

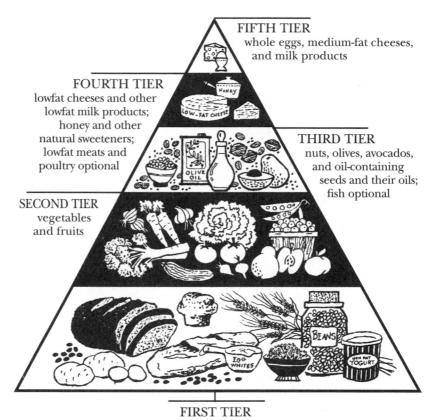

FIFTH TIER
whole eggs, medium-fat cheeses,
and milk products

FOURTH TIER
lowfat cheeses and other
lowfat milk products;
honey and other
natural sweeteners;
lowfat meats and
poultry optional

THIRD TIER
nuts, olives, avocados,
and oil-containing
seeds and their oils;
fish optional

SECOND TIER
vegetables
and fruits

FIRST TIER
whole grains, beans, nonfat or very lowfat yogurts
and milk products, and egg whites

cancer survivors and it is in agreement with the way diets are designed in this book (see Figure 4.1).

You can use the Superpyramid as a guideline at anytime during your recovery cycle to decide how often to eat a certain food. The foods on the two bottom tiers should be the foundation of your diet, the foods on the third tier should be used to complement these foods, and the foods on the fourth and fifth tiers should only be used in great moderation.

Figure 4.2   *The Cancer Survivor's Pyramid*

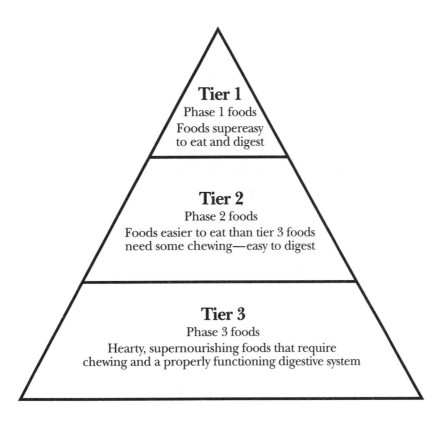

Tier 1
Phase 1 foods
Foods supereasy
to eat and digest

Tier 2
Phase 2 foods
Foods easier to eat than tier 3 foods
need some chewing—easy to digest

Tier 3
Phase 3 foods
Hearty, supernourishing foods that require
chewing and a properly functioning digestive system

A NEW KIND OF PYRAMID

The Cancer Survivor's Pyramid shows you how certain foods fit in with the various special needs of the cancer survivor (see Figure 4.2).

Look at it as a new tool to help you. Do not try to compare it with the Superpyramid or other pyramids. It is not based on how often you should eat certain foods (like the USDA *Food Guide Pyramid*), but rather it places the great healing and protective foods on three different tiers according to different recovery phases and how easy or difficult those kinds of foods generally are to eat.

HOW TO USE THE CANCER SURVIVOR'S PYRAMID

First of all, identify what phase of recovery you feel you are in. Remember that you may find that you change phases daily, depending upon how you feel. Be flexible about choosing foods from the different tiers at any given time. The ultimate goal is to make *Tier 3* the foundation of your diet whenever possible.

Where Are You Right Now?

Generally speaking, there are three phases, starting with *Phase 1*, that some cancer survivors experience. You may or may not have any problems, so the best advice is to aim for the highest phase you feel comfortable at, at any given time.

Phase 1   This usually occurs during treatment, and may be one of the most difficult times for you—though the positive side is that it will most likely be temporary. During this period, food choices and methods of preparation are crucial. You may not feel hungry, and your digestive system may not be quite right. Even the thought and sight of food may not be welcome. But if you don't get enough food, you will feel tired, lethargic, and apathetic, and possibly be unable to get around. In addition, your body's ability to rebuild itself will be slowed and could even be halted. You must be sure to get enough to eat and that you eat real food—although this may be supplemented by liquid meals (page 83) whenever needed. If you do this, you will likely find yourself better able to handle and cope with any unpleasant aftereffects that may occur. And moreover, you will be enhancing the repair process and helping to bolster your resistance to future

In a Nutshell

Use the Cancer Survivor's Pyramid to guide your food choices, choosing your guiding tier according to the phase of your recovery. Use the Superpyramid to further learn about the relative need for various types of foods.

illness. *This first phase needs **Supereasy**, supernourishing, perhaps even sippable foods that are easy to eat and digest and made from appealing wholesome ingredients.*

Phase 2   On the path to healing and rebuilding, some of you may enter a *Phase 2*, while others go directly to *Phase 3*. Here, in *Phase 2*, you are beginning to feel better or even well. The chemotherapy or other treatment is over, or you have become adjusted and feel more normal, but you are still not yourself completely. Your body is spending a lot of its energy to restore itself to health, and it must also continue to work to protect itself from recurrence or future illness. *This phase needs **Easy** foods for digestion, but usually not Supereasy or sippable foods, that are still supernourishing, with fairly mild flavors and soft textures.*

Phase 3   Finally, all or most of the treatment aftereffects are a thing of the past. You feel that your appetite is now normal. You are not as tired, and are able to be more physically active. Your mouth is comfortable with chewing; you can swallow; and your digestive tract is back to normal or nearly normal. This is the time or times in between treatment sessions, or after you have completed all your treatment cycles, that you should be making the foods of the optimum diet central to your eating. *Phase 3* is when you will be able to enjoy the wholesome flavors and textures that accompany *Hearty,* supernourishing foods.

Choosing Foods from the Pyramid Tiers by Recovery Phase

We know that some foods like mashed, peeled potatoes are easy to eat and digest, while foods like kidney beans are heartier and take more work to digest—which is sometimes too trying when you are not feeling well. Use the tiers to quickly find the right foods for you at any given time; they are arranged by ease of eating and handling by the body.

Tier 1: The Top Tier—The Gentlest of All   *Tier 1* is at the top of the Cancer Survivor's Pyramid and is the smallest. Here we find only those foods that are **Supereasy** to eat. They are optimum choices for those short periods of times when you're feeling the least well, are experiencing difficulty swallowing, and have little or no appetite or are having digestive problems, which may occur during *Phase 1*. The choices on this tier are extremely important since they provide you with vital energy and nutrients. You should aim to walk down to *Tier 2* as soon as possible. Then to *Tier 3,* where you literally have a lot of space to move around and a wide variety of choices.

On *Tier 1* we find *liquid* foods—many of which come from the earth or are combined with high quality animal proteins. We use the term *sippable* for these kinds of foods. Some examples are:

Super Sippables (see page 83) of all sorts
Thin cereal gruels
Thin purees of fruits and vegetables, especially from potatoes,
    sweet potatoes, winter squash, and carrots
Fruit and vegetable juices (usually strained)
Milk and milk drinks
Teas
Special liquid supplements or meals

Tier 2: The Middle Tier—In-Between Foods   *Tier 2* is designed for the times when you need foods that are *Easy* to digest, but you are able to chew or handle some soft foods in your mouth. Foods still need to be gentle on your digestive tract. Many of these food choices are the same as in *Tier 3,* but are milder in flavor, softer in texture, and are easier to eat and digest. The only reason some foods are excluded (like cooked dry beans, tempeh, whole nuts, and some fruits and vegetables) is because they are harder to eat and/or digest.

On *Tier 2* we find foods such as:

Cooked dry beans, which have been put through a ricer to remove the skins; red lentils, and tofu.

Just about all the grains. (You should use, whenever possible, *whole* grains like oats, barley, millet, stone-ground cornmeal, couscous, and wheat germ. But when the situation calls for it, pastas and grains made from refined white flour are OK to use occasionally.)

Good fats such as olive and sesame oils, avocados, nut and seed butters. (These are important for adding flavor and valuable antioxidants.)

Soft, cooked vegetables, especially cooked greens, carrots, winter squashes, and potatoes. (Peeling or seeding helps to make these easier to eat and digest.) *Note:* Broccoli and cabbage family vegetables are usually not easily digested, so use is limited—but don't bypass them if they sound good to you and you think you can handle them.

Peeled and seed-free, fresh, dried, and/or cooked fruits—especially avocados, bananas, citrus, mangos, papayas, peaches, apricots, nectarines, plums, pears, pumpkins, and raisins. *Note:* Berries with seeds and melons are usually more difficult to digest.

Nonfat (or 1% lowfat) milk and milk products (like yogurt, ricotta and cottage cheese, and kefir).

Eggs (or just egg whites, if cholesterol concerns you).

Finally, fragrant and flavorful herbs and spices, used liberally and frequently. *Note:* During *Phase 2* of recovery, powdered versions that still give you some flavor may be more easily handled than leaves.

Tier 3: The Bottom Tier—A Cornucopia of Hearty and Wholesome Foods Tier 3 is very spacious and supports the entire structure of the Cancer Survivor's Pyramid. This tier is for you after you have fully recovered from treatment, usually *Phase 3,* or for periods during treatment when you feel totally normal and hungry, ready to digest anything. It comprises all the best **Hearty, supernourishing** choices you can make. These foods must be the cornerstone of your diet—and your family's too. The cornucopia of foods on this tier includes items that are also found on the upper tiers, but which can be enjoyed with little or no change, as hearty and rich in texture as they come. The *Tier 3* foods usually require a normal ability to chew and swallow, and a properly functioning digestive system. On this tier we find:

Cooked dry beans, lentils, split peas, and soybean products (such as tofu and tempeh), which fill in the need for superb protein as well as energy, fiber, vitamins, minerals, and many protective substances.

Whole grains and good sources of fiber—like whole grain breads and pastas, brown and wild rice, hulled barley, couscous, wheat germ, and bulgur, with their abundance of energy, protein, vitamins, and minerals.

Good fats such as olive and sesame oils, avocados, and nut and seed butters. (These are important for adding flavor and valuable antioxidants.)

Fresh, cooked, or dried fruits and vegetables of all colors and textures, prepared as you prefer.

Nonfat (or 1% lowfat) milk and milk products (like yogurt, ricotta and cottage cheese, and kefir) to help supply calcium and high quality protein.

Eggs (or just egg whites, if cholesterol concerns you).

Finally, fragrant and flavorful herbs and spices, used liberally and frequently.

Chapter 5

HANDLING SPECIAL SITUATIONS

THIS CHAPTER COVERS SPECIFIC HEALTH AND DIET CON-
siderations. You may choose to read only the sections that pertain
to your situation or problem. If you do not have any eating problems or aftereffects during or soon after treatment, you can skip
this chapter and go on to Chapter 6.

EATING PROBLEMS DURING TREATMENT

Drugs and radiation therapy are often so good at destroying
tumor cells that they also damage healthy cells vital to our well
being. Cells that reproduce very rapidly in the body, like the
cells of the intestine and blood, are extremely sensitive to cancer treatments. The results are poor appetite and digestion, and,
often, nausea as well. The decrease in the number of white
blood cells results in lowered resistance to infections, and the
reduction in the number of red blood cells makes you feel tired
and weak.

The bright side is that most cancer survivors do not have this
problem for very long after treatment has been completed, and

some may have no eating problems at all. According to the National Institute of Health, an agency of the Federal Government, "Side effects of cancer treatment vary from patient to patient. The part of the body being treated, length of treatment, and the dose of treatment also affect whether side effects will occur . . . The good news is that only about one-third of cancer patients have side effects during treatment."

Still, nothing takes away more from the enjoyment of eating than not feeling well. In extreme cases, the total physiological or psychological rejection of foods can result in vomiting soon after eating. A sore mouth or difficulty in chewing and swallowing can also contribute to discomfort.

Remember that while you are going through treatment or experiencing its aftereffects, the healing process continues to go on and what you eat at this time plays a vital role in replenishing your body's nutrient stores and in rebuilding your strength. You must avoid any food with possible negative effects and eat plenty of foods rich in protective, building nutrients. While this is true at any stage of your recovery and even when you are completely back to normal, it is even more true while treatment is in progress. If you have a poor appetite and you find food unappealing, this is the time to get the most out of every little bite that you put into your mouth.

After the end of a treatment cycle, it may take a few days or weeks to get totally back to normal. In this period you may continue to use *Supereasy* foods and slowly begin to add *Easy* foods; eventually you will begin to eat more and more of the *Hearty* recipes you'll find in this book. Remember that when you are back to normal, you should continue to eat as many protective foods as possible—this sounds logical and yet many people tend to forget the need for supernutrition once they feel well again. As a cancer survivor, a good diet based on superprotective foods is more important to you than to anyone else.

In a Nutshell

Foods and recipes that we define as Supereasy are a crucial part of the diet of the cancer survivor during treatment, if there are any eating problems. These foods have to be easy to eat, easy to digest, and extremely kind to the digestive system.

WHAT CAN I DO WHEN I'M FEELING GOOD?

Even if during treatment you have difficult periods, there will be times when you'll feel well. During these times the key is to learn the most you can about yourself and what you may be able eat when you are low and weak. Planning ahead will give you resources to draw from, and solutions that you handpicked yourself and that you know will work. You will then be able to meet the difficult situations head on. Here are four key things that you can do when you are feeling strong and able so you'll be ready for any periods when you might feel low and weak:

Make a List of Your Favorite Foods and Beverages

The first thing to do is to find out which foods you love from the optimum foods lists of Chapter 2, so you can make them your first choices during a not-so-hungry period. *Make a list of these foods and keep it in a place where you can find or see it easily when you do not feel like doing much.* You may want to post your list on your refrigerator door or write it on your kitchen calendar. Use the sample pantry list at the end of this book and use your highlighter to mark the foods you like best or that you might like to try. When you can, buy some of these foods and keep them as staples in the pantry so they will be handy. This works especially well for dry beans, nuts, seeds, pastas, brown rice, and dried fruits. Boldly mark the recipes in this book that you like.

Double Your Efficiency

For some cancer survivors periods of fatigue are predictable, such as after a treatment session. Try to pinpoint these and identify them when or if they occur. Then identify the foods that would be easiest for you to prepare and eat. A few foods that are the simplest to prepare and eat include:

Super Sippables (pages 83–97)
Simply Miso soup (page 118)
Pasta in Brodo di Casa (page 121)
Fifty Ways to Have Hot Grains (page 188)
Sweet Cooked Apple (page 198)

Also, when you are feeling well, prepare double batches of recipes that sound good to you and freeze them for reheating when you don't feel so well. *See Appendix A at the end of this book that lists recipes that freeze well (page 213).*

Make Food and Meals as Engaging as You Can

Before you lose your appetite make notes to yourself about what makes a meal most pleasurable and enticing to you. Some cancer survivors find a special kind of lighting inspiring, like candle-light, as well as playing some good music, using special china, crystal, or silver, or simply putting fresh flowers on the table. Do something that will make you feel special or bring back happy memories. Often these psychological devices have not only a favorable mental effect, but also a direct physiological effect that helps to stimulate appetite.

Become aware of textures, flavors, and even colors that tend to stimulate your appetite. For example, the contrast of red and blue berries with white yogurt or the texture of a grain mixed with raisins and nuts are appetizing and appealing to many people. Also be aware of those things you don't like, so you'll be clear about what to stay away from.

Accept and Enjoy Support from Family and Friends

People do like to help out. Be honest and tell your friends and family how you feel and what you would like. Make photocopies of the **pantry** list and give one to whomever is helping you, or if you do your own shopping, bring it with you to the store.

MORE GENERAL HINTS FOR HANDLING TROUBLESOME AFTEREFFECTS

Aftereffects of treatment can range from episodes of lack of appetite, an off-sense of taste and smell, mouth or throat soreness, chewing or swallowing difficulties, nausea and vomiting, constipation or diarrhea, or even just being simply too tired to want to bother with eating. Here are some hints:

Dig out your list and concentrate on those favorite optimum foods, as they may help stimulate your appetite.

Keep simple and easy to eat foods handy: a chilled fruit nectar, some fresh soft fruits like peaches in the summer or ripe pears in the winter, perhaps some dried fruits like raisins, or *Juice Cubies* (page 86).

Heat a quick cup of miso in the microwave (page 118).

Eat several small portions of food made from favorite foods throughout the day (even better, eat at structured times), instead of a few big meals.

Grab a small portion of yogurt and sprinkle it with wheat germ.

Make your eating environment as special as you can.

Dig out those meals that you froze and reheat them.

Keep the foods you love in sight.

Let someone else do the cooking (this is a good time to accept and enjoy the support of family and friends).

FOOD IDEAS FOR FEELING BETTER	☐ Dried fruit like sun-dried raisins ☐ Chilled fruit juices, nectars, or smoothies ☐ Miso or other soothing soups—throw in a few tofu cubes for protein ☐ Pureed or other soft fruits and vegetables, like applesauce, fresh peaches, bananas, a fruit whip, mashed potatoes, sweet potatoes, or carrots (seasoned or plain) ☐ Thin or thick, hot, whole grain cereal with honey or syrup ☐ Yogurt with wheat germ and honey

Now it's time to discuss some specific aftereffects of cancer treatment, with foods and ideas to help you get through.

NAUSEA

A common aftereffect of treatment or even the illness itself is the unsettling of the digestive tract. It's a good idea to keep track of the time when it occurs, and then, when possible, to try to modify your food choices or your schedule. If the nausea is extreme, don't hesitate to ask your health professional for advice or medication. Here are a few practical ideas:

Eat small amounts often and slowly.

Maintain a relaxed and comfortable environment; stress and anxiety can add to nausea.

Wear loose-fitting clothes to help you feel more relaxed.

Rest after meals.

Try to sit up for about an hour after eating.

Keep liquid intake with meals to a minimum. Instead drink or sip liquids throughout the day. Too much liquid with a meal can make your stomach feel full and bloated, adding to the discomfort. Some people feel that using a straw to drink helps.

Try foods and beverages at room temperature or chilled. They usually have less aroma or flavor than very warm foods, which can trigger nauseous feelings.

Try not to eat one to two hours before treatment, if you've noticed that nausea occurs afterwards. A common spice, ginger (page 30), may also help with nausea. Try mixing half of a teaspoon of ground ginger into tea or juice, and sipping it slowly. Or make a plain ginger tea flavored with honey (page 95). You might even try drinking ginger tea a half-hour to one hour before treatment if you usually experience nausea after a treatment session. Ask your health professional first before doing this.

<table>
<tr><td>SOME SPECIFIC
FOOD IDEAS TO
TRY</td><td>☐ Dry toast or crackers (can be helpful for morning nausea if eaten before getting up)
☐ Small bites of plain yogurt or yogurt cheese on small cubes of whole grain bread
☐ Ice chips or Juice Cubies (page 86)
☐ Bland, soft fruits like peaches or applesauce
☐ Plain mashed potatoes or cooked carrot sticks
☐ Popsicles made by putting popsicle sticks into cups of yogurt, then covering and freezing them.
☐ Mild, room temperature chamomile or peppermint teas</td></tr>
</table>

Avoid your favorite foods as you may inadvertently create a dis-
   like or aversion to them!
Leave out fatty, greasy foods.

VOMITING

Some immunotherapy and radiation therapies may cause you to
experience vomiting. This can occur in response to gas in your
stomach or bowel, motion, or even food odors. Vomiting can be
very serious if it is persistent, resulting in the further depletion of
your already weak condition. You can become dehydrated and
lose the nutrients that you need so badly from vomiting. Whenever vomiting lasts more than a few days, contact your health
professional. They may recommend some medicine to help you.
Here are some additional ideas:

One of the most common and useful strategies for vomiting
when it occurs only infrequently, is not to try to force yourself to
eat or drink until the episode has passed or is under control.

Try only very tiny amounts of liquids, like tiny sips of something that is bland or light in flavor (like room temperature
diluted juice, lukewarm miso broth, or ginger tea—page 95). Try
to suck on ice chips. Continue doing this until you feel better

and more normal. Then gradually increase your intake of liquids as you feel better.

Many people find that their vomiting is helped when they start with clear liquids, followed by heartier, more nutrient-packed ones. When they feel better, they add more soft and regular foods as tolerance returns. The following sections offer some ideas for foods during these times.

Clear Liquids That Are Very Easy on the Digestive Tract

Mild teas, plain or with honey (chamomile, ginger, and peppermint teas appear to help with nausea and vomiting).

Mineral waters, carbonated or plain.

Miso broth or other mild, vegetable-based broths.

Fruit juices or nectars, without pulp or strained; mild vegetable juice (like diluted carrot juice).

Frozen, mild flavored fruit juice or nectar cubes (pour nectar into ice cube tray and freeze).

Heartier, More Nutrient-Packed Liquids

When you're feeling better, you can choose some heartier foods, sometimes called full liquid meals or diets:

Pureed soups at room temperature. Try carrot, potato, or winter squash soup that has been blended and thinned with milk.

Well cooked cereals, thinned with milk; top with plain or fruit-flavored yogurt if you can tolerate it. Avoid fruit pieces in yogurt.

Soft or baked custards without fruit pieces.

Fresh or frozen, nonfat or lowfat (1%), plain or fruit-flavored yogurts without fruit pieces; or kefir.

Juice, nectars and thin fruit purees, other drinks and smoothies (pages 85–96).

Mashed, cooked vegetables (like potatoes, carrots, sweet potatoes,

Clear Liquid Menu Ideas for a Day

Meal	Menu
Morning	Apricot nectar
	Warm, mild tea with honey
Noon	Miso soup
	Strawberry guava juice
Evening	Miso or vegetable broth
	Carrot juice
Snacks	Peach nectar cubes
	Tea with honey
	Apricot pineapple nectar

Full Liquid Menu Ideas for a Day

Meal	Menu
Morning	Hi-energy soy milk cocoa (page 91)
	Cooked, thinned polenta with honey mixed in
	Warm, mild tea with honey
Noon	Mashed and thinned sweet potatoes
	Miso broth
	Applesauce and pear puree
	Papaya-pineapple juice
	Warm, mild tea with honey
Evening	Puree of Fresh Fennel soup (page 112)
	Mashed Simply Squash with pure maple syrup (page 172)
	Fruit Whip with Ricotta Cheese (page 192)
	Warm, mild tea with honey
Snacks	Almond milk
	Any fruit nectar
	Baked Yogurt Honey Custard
	Any Super Sippable (pages 83–98)

and winter squash) thinned with milk or yogurt to a thick puree; can be plain or seasoned.

Medical liquid meals prepared from purified ingredients (page 20).

Soft foods

Soft foods are for the times when your body is ready for solid foods but still needs a gentle touch. These kinds of foods are generally easier to eat and digest when your mouth, throat, esophagus, or stomach are not doing well.

Well cooked cereals (whole grain if possible), topped with yogurt and soft fruits.

Eggs, like soft scrambles, soft or baked custards (pages 99–107).

Fresh or frozen yogurts with or without fruit pieces, yogurt cheese, regular milk, kefir, or buttermilk.

Soft, *real* whole wheat breads without seeds or nuts (trim crust, if desired).

All pastas and noodles (preferably whole wheat, but 100 percent durum wheat semolina flour is OK), peeled potatoes and sweet potatoes, rice (brown is best), and millet.

Smooth nut butters like almond and sesame butter.

All juices, nectars, and cooked fruits; limit raw fruit to bananas, avocados, and soft melons (if tolerated).

All cooked vegetables except those that tend to be hard to digest; these include vegetables found in the cruciferous family (these include broccoli, cauliflower, cabbages, greens like kale, collard, or turnip greens), the onion family, and cooked dry beans, peas, and lentils.

DIARRHEA

Diarrhea may be due to many causes and is often the result of the therapy on the digestive system. The loose, watery stools of diarrhea can result in loss of vitamins, minerals, and water; in extreme cases, it can lead to dehydration and increased risk of infection. Whenever diarrhea lasts more than a few days or is severe, be sure to contact your health professional. Here are some tips for occasional episodes:

Soft Foods Menu Idea for a Day

Meal	Menu
Morning	Incredible Versatile Eggs (page 101)
	Oatmeal with cooked peaches
	soft, whole wheat toast with almond butter
	Warm, mild tea with honey
Noon	Potato Soup with Spinach Ribbons (page 122)
	Soft, whole wheat roll spread with Yogurt Cheese (page 210)
	Banana with nut butter
	Pear-peach nectar
	Warm, mild tea with honey
Evening	Linguine with Asparagus, Portobello Mushrooms, and Ginger (page 139)
	Soft, whole wheat bread
	Carrot juice
	Sweet Cooked Apple (page 198)
	Warm, mild tea with honey
Snacks	Fruit juice/nectar
	Cooked fruits (peeled, and with no seeds)
	Almond milk (page 90)
	Plain custard/pudding
	Any Super Sippable (pages 83–97)

Drink lots of room temperature liquids to help prevent dehydration. If possible, drink on a schedule and make sure you get a glass of fluid at least once an hour. Focus on nutrient-packed liquids, especially those high in sodium and potassium that won't cause diarrhea. Good high potassium foods include peach and apricot nectars, oranges, and bananas.

Try a well-baked apple or applesauce made with the skin. These contain pectin, which helps retain water and improve stool consistency.

Temporarily decrease your fiber intake (normally you want to eat plenty of fiber to stay healthy). Try yogurts, pasta and noodles made from 100% durum wheat semolina flour, cooked eggs, smooth nut butters, and, temporarily, breads made from refined flour without seeds or nuts. (Go back to your whole grain breads as soon as you can!) Limit use of any other fruits and stay away from raw vegetables and fruits, very spicy or highly seasoned foods, and very hot or very cold foods and beverages. Also limit your caffeine intake for the time being.

CONSTIPATION

As constipation is the opposite of diarrhea, the treatment is in a way the opposite, too. The key to preventing it is fiber. The digestive tract can be slowed down by the medicines you are taking, the stress you are experiencing, and the kinds of foods you are eating. Here are some tips—but if nothing works, and before you take any laxatives, contact your health professional.

Every day drink plenty of liquids. If possible schedule your drinking: Be sure you get a glass of fluid at least once an hour. Focus on nutrient-packed liquids like fresh fruit and vegetable juices. Don't forget good plain water!

Focus on high fiber foods. Whole grains—breads, rice, cereals, and pastas—contain the kind of fibers especially helpful in preventing constipation. But don't discount fresh fruits and vegetables with skins and peels. Cooked dry beans, peas, and lentils—as well as dried fruits, such as sun-dried raisins—are also beneficial.

Add unprocessed wheat bran to hot cereals and yogurt.

Try to be physically active each day.

A reminder: When you increase your fiber intake you must be sure to drink plenty of fluids. Increasing fiber without also increasing fluid intake can actually have the opposite effect and contribute to constipation or, in rare cases, even intestinal blockage.

WHEN FOOD TASTES OR SMELLS FUNNY

You may find that favorite foods suddenly don't taste like they did. You may notice that you have a numbness or metallic or bitter taste in your mouth, and that some flavors are harder to recognize. This can occur during certain cancer treatments, especially during or soon after chemotherapy. Do you find that sweet things taste either sweeter or less sweet and that some foods taste saltier or not salty enough? Do foods have little or no taste? These are just some of the sensations we have heard about. Here are some tips to handle these situations:

When foods have less taste: Use tart foods like oranges or lemons as a seasoning; and more flavorful seasonings like curry powder, garlic, or pepper.

When taste is exaggerated or foods smell funny: Try cold or room temperature foods which may taste better as flavors and aromas are usually less noticeable. Try chilled soups, cold sandwiches, and mild fresh fruits and vegetables, like kiwis and jicama.

In either case: Use a prepared liquid meal that appeals to you. If you feel like it, blend in some fresh juice, fruit nectar, or, if you use a blender or food processor, add a banana or other fruit.

CHEWING OR SWALLOWING DIFFICULTIES

Tenderness and soreness in the mouth and throat are not uncommon and are usually directly related to treatment. These aftereffects can challenge even the most stalwart cancer survivors and make getting enough food seem like an enormous undertaking. This is the time to intensify your efforts to get as much nourishment as you can, since getting it down will take effort. Some ideas that work are:

Try Very Soft or Thick Liquid Foods

Choose nutrient-rich shakes and smoothies made with Super-Foods like yogurt, tofu, fruit and vegetable juices.

Puree or blenderize potatoes, carrots, yams, and soups; they usually work well. Again you may use a liquid meal.

Soak whole grain breads in warm milk; make a bread pudding; dunk a slice of bread in a cup of tea prepared with some milk and honey.

Eat custards or scrambled eggs with tofu (see page 99).

Try Different Ways of Eating

Use a straw or drink from a cup instead of using a spoon.

Eat foods that are room temperature or cold; they may be easier to swallow than hot foods. Hot foods can be troublesome; while cold foods may be better tolerated.

Frozen Juice Cubies (see page 86) or bars often help to numb the tissues and also help to increase your fluid intake.

Add sauces or olive oil to foods to ease swallowing.

Don't get stuck in a boring routine.

CHANGES IN FOOD TOLERANCE

Become aware of what you can tolerate. It's important not to forget that your tolerances and preferences can change overnight. Acid foods like salad dressings and certain spices (like pepper, chile powder, and cloves) can be irritating to the mouth: Use them sparingly or eliminate them for the time being. Go back to them when you feel better.

BODY WEIGHT CHANGES

Weight Gain

Gaining weight may be due to various medicines, decreased physical activity, fluid retention, or even increased appetite. Do not go on any "weight loss diet" that is not meant for a person recovering from cancer. If you have questions about a particular diet, seek advice from your health professional. In general, a diet that is based on whole plant foods, and low in animal products and animal fats, is also the first step to weight control.

Weight Loss

Whenever you take in fewer calories (energy) than your body needs or you don't retain the calories you take in, weight loss will occur. Some of the common aftereffects of treatment, like loss of appetite, vomiting, and diarrhea, can contribute to weight loss. First, when you are losing weight, try to determine what's contributing to it. Are you eating much less because of some treatment aftereffect? Are you frequently experiencing digestive tract problems like vomiting and diarrhea? If so, try some of the tips offered here. If you are eating less, for any reason, here are some foods to add calories:

Wheat germ: Add to cooked cereals and casseroles; try blending it into smoothies.

Add honey, pure maple syrup, or molasses to cereals, milk and other drinks, fruits, yogurt, and bread.

Add nonfat dry milk powder to drinks, casseroles, and custards.

Spread nut butters on bread; add to cooked whole grain cereals.

Use olive oil in salads, and as a topping for vegetables and bread.

Add dried fruits to cereals, cooked vegetables like carrots, sweet potatoes and winter squash; mix with nut butter and spread on bread.

Add hard cooked eggs to salads, vegetables, and casseroles.

Beat raw eggs into potatoes and vegetable purees, being sure to continue cooking the food until the eggs are done to avoid bacterial infection.

Enjoy different kinds of nuts as snacks or a part of snacks; add them to cereals, desserts, casseroles, rice, and pasta; top vegetables with them.

Use sweet potatoes in place of white potatoes for added calories as well as for their high phytochemical content. Eat them baked or boiled, hot or cold from the refrigerator. Cook with honey, syrup, or molasses.

Drink fruit nectars, smoothies, or protein shakes as snacks.

A CANCER SURVIVOR'S STORY

Jim is a successful senior vice president of a major pharmaceutical corporation. In his early forties, Jim is very health-conscious and athletic and has run a number of marathons and the San Francisco Bay to Breakers race many times. To his dismay, as he had never smoked, Jim learned that he had a lung tumor four years ago. The cancer growth was removed surgically and Jim lost half a lung. This slowed down his athletic performance but still allowed him to do all activities. As there was still a chance that some cancer cells could spread to other parts of his body, chemotherapy and radiation were recommended after the surgery. Jim is now leading a normal and full working life, with an occasional interruption for a treatment session. He has learned to handle all phases of treatment and recovery well, and he describes his experiences in his own words.

"During my treatment I went through two phases. First, after the initiation of the chemotherapy, I went through a period of time when I felt quite sick and did not feel like eating. There was nausea and sometimes vomiting. Some medication I was given helped prevent some of these unwanted effects, but I still had this initial response. Then later there was a second phase of the treatment period when I just felt tired and run down. The reason was most likely that many of my blood cells were destroyed together with the bad cancer cells.

"In the early days of treatment I did well with easy-to-take liquid meals, soups, and what you call in this book "sippable" foods—all easy to digest. I often added a banana or other fruits to my shakes. Their fiber helped me to prevent the constipation that a fiber-free liquid meal can cause and we all know fruits contain

In a Nutshell

Remember: The times when you are weak and do not feel like eating are the times when you need the energy, the proteins, and all the protective factors of foods more than ever!

many protective factors. Another advantage, to me, of these liquid, drinkable foods was that I could consume them in a short sitting and be reassured that I was getting my nutrients and calories. When rushed at the office, I felt I could still get my proper diet in one of these drinkable foods, rather than getting my energy from some potato chips or high fat, low fiber cookies or some junk food.

"When the major problems caused by the chemotherapy subsided and I just felt tired but not sick, I tried to eat more whole plant foods like grains and vegetables as well as fruits. My wife prepared lots of vegetable-based dishes, like carrots and spinach. Ornate dishes, even if low in fat, did not appeal to me at all during any stages of chemotherapy or in the early days that followed. I just wanted simple foods somewhat bland in taste and easy-to-eat. In phase two, my energy came from pasta, noodles, rice, and potatoes . . . there was no way I could go out to dinner with friends and try to eat what they ate.

"These days, when the intermittent treatments are behind me and I am in phase three (page 41), I begin to feel like eating more ornate, spicy, and flavorful foods, more sauces, and can again use tomato sauce on my pasta. I again enjoy normal foods. We as a family always try to eat the best possible diet to prevent disease and possible cancer recurrence, a diet higher in plant foods, fiber, and antioxidants—and low in animal fats. In all phases of recovery, I always eat, as much as possible, a plant-based diet: I am not a vegetarian, but the foundation of the diet of the 'cancer survivor' must be plant foods."

Chapter 6

BEYOND FOOD

THERE IS MORE TO THE RECOVERY FROM CANCER AND the prevention of future recurrence than food. We all know it, and yet we all tend to forget that health is a complex interaction of food, environmental factors, and physical activity. There are things we must do and there are things we must avoid. It sounds simple, but most of us forget it too often. In our modern complex world exposure to stress, noise, pollution, and radiation are all around us, much more than just a century ago. Let's just mention a few.

On the "do" list we find:
physical activity
proper rest
positive attitude
stress reduction

On the "don't" list we find:
smoking and smoke
stress, mental and physical
polluted air and car fumes
exposure to toxic chemicals
radiation

During and soon after treatment, the effects of both positive and negative factors are of extreme importance, but they should not be forgotten after you are back to normal. Just like proper protective foods and avoiding negative foods, they will be crucial for the rest of your life.

PHYSICAL ACTIVITY

There is no complete health without physical activity. The human body was meant to be active. Loss of muscle, what scientists call *atrophy,* happens very rapidly with inactivity, and this is what happens to people in wheelchairs or after a prolonged bed rest because of a major injury or illness. It has been known for a long time that the body goes into a negative balance during prolonged rest: More of certain nutrients go out than in, no matter how much you consume of that nutrient. Two of the major nutrients that are affected are protein and calcium, both of which are vital to good recovery and health.

Whenever you feel well enough, do something physical. Walk, stretch, lift some light weights. Check with your health professional before getting involved in intense activities if you have any doubts. But after, when you are back to normal, do some intense activities as frequently as possible.

The body does better if you do some of each of the three basic types of exercises:

1. Aerobics, like walking, climbing a hill, jogging, bicycling, and swimming
2. Stretching, like many yoga exercises
3. Weight lifting, which does not mean heavy weight lifting, but moderate and as fits your pre-cancer strength

The Exercise Pyramid is a useful tool for understanding how all types of exercises fit in the picture of health (see Figure 5.1).

In a Nutshell
This is just a short list of key points to make us realize that we need not just the right food, but also that we need to consider our total lifestyle to do all we can to get well and stay well.

Figure 5.1 *The Exercise Pyramid*

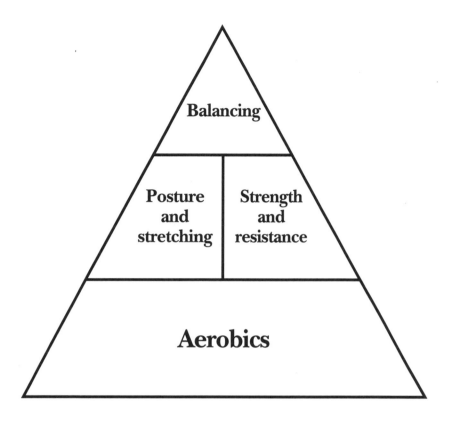

Here's how it's designed: On the bottom tier are the aerobic activities, which should be the foundation of your exercise plan. On the second tier are stretching and posturing exercises, plus strength or resistance exercises such as moderate weight lifting. Tier three, the smallest tier, features balancing activities such as walking on a balance beam. This will help you develop body awareness and confidence when doing other physical activities.

PROPER REST AND AVOIDING STRESS

Proper rest and avoiding stress are just as important as physical activity. Special techniques often help. For example, many people find massage by a trained therapist an excellent way to reduce stress. The modern world is full of noises, like those of car engines. We are surrounded by radio, TV, fast moving events, traffic jams, and a whole list of other stressful events that could fill pages. We can't avoid them all, but we can do our best to minimize their impact or decrease our exposure to some of them.

It is especially important to avoid physical stresses, as well as mental stresses, in the early days of recovery. We have talked about the value of exercise, but that does not mean that you should try to become involved in activities that are overly taxing. It is difficult to generalize when physical activity becomes a harmful stress, as it depends on what your fitness was before your cancer treatments—you must be the judge—but the early recovery days are not the time for extremes.

Make a special effort to have normal and sufficient sleep. Take a nap in the daytime if you are tired. If you are going back to work, try to find a few quiet moments for an occasional rest, just as you would for some physical activity.

One last word: A major, overlooked cause of stress is travel, especially airplane travel, as is any change of time zones greater than an hour or two. Sleep patterns are upset and some people sleep poorly for a few days at their new destination. Avoid such travel if you can in the early days of recovery.

THE POWER OF THE MIND AND OF POSITIVE ATTITUDES

The power of the mind is too often overlooked in modern Western societies, which are so focused on hard, biological facts.

Dr. Thomas Delbanco of the Harvard School of Medicine, in an interview in Bill Moyers' book, *Healing and the Mind,* admits that: ". . . I know more about the body than the mind . . . and that's what we have learned in medical school, ninety-five percent body and five percent mind." But the mind is the controlling center of our body, and because it does have a crucial effect on health and disease, it is becoming more and more accepted in Western medicine. As Dr. Ron Anderson, a physician who has held major positions in the Texas medical world, says in another interview in the same book: ". . . if you do not understand the mind-body connection [of a patient], you start off on the wrong premise." Asian medicine and religions have long accepted the power of a total peaceful focusing on a given topic—for the cancer survivor, this means faith in recovery and healing—and there is much wisdom to be learned from these medical traditions.

As a cancer survivor, you must believe in recovery as, if nothing else, this belief will bring you the courage to do all you can to get completely well. A positive attitude is what some people call "faith." A peaceful period when you isolate yourself from the world is what may be called "meditation." Think of this: *The fact that you are reading this book is a sign of a positive attitude.*

SMOKING, POLLUTED AIR, AND CAR FUMES

In the early 1980s, in the autopsy room of the Stanford School of Medicine, medical students examined the body of a woman who had died of lung cancer as a consequence of smoking. Her history was tragic: She had had one lung removed and had survived the surgery well, but as soon as she was out of the hospital, she began to smoke again. Later new tumors appeared in the other lung and death was the outcome.

Remember that smoke in general, not just tobacco smoke, and its products are cancer-producing agents. Back centuries ago, one of the first correlations of environment and cancer was found when a British physician linked cancer in chimney sweepers to their inhaling and being in daily contact with the residues of burning coal in the chimneys of London. Smoke from a barbecue is cancer-producing, as is tobacco smoking. It's amazing some people still doubt that smoke is bad!

Fumes from cars and from gasoline are to be avoided too. Avoid jogging on a road with heavy traffic, as you'll inhale even more car fumes while jogging than if you were walking. If you have had cancer, avoid all fumes and tobacco much more so than anyone else. You may be particularly sensitive to them for whatever reason, something in your genes or some event in early childhood.

RADIATION

Radiation from computer monitors and cellular phones tends to damage cells. Avoid regular use of cellular phones; use them as an occasional and often valuable necessity. Don't sit to the side of a computer monitor: Manufacturers are doing a nice job to reduce radiation from monitors, but remember that a lot of it comes out from the side. In an office, try not to sit next to someone else's desk with the side of their monitor close to you.

Excessive exposure to the sun for long periods and especially sunburn can also do damage. This should be of special concern to very fair-skinned people, who often come from a Nordic ancestry.

EXPOSURE TO TOXIC CHEMICALS AND DRUGS

This may apply only to certain professions or activities, such as a scientist or technician in a laboratory where powerful chemicals are used daily. Some of these are compounds with outright cancer-producing properties, while others may weaken the immune system, opening the door to other cancer-producing agents. If your profession calls for the use of toxic substances, you must be extra careful when in contact with these chemicals.

If you use sprays or poisons in your garden or house, be extra careful as, just like with smoke, you may be more sensitive than someone who has not had cancer. Avoid inhaling any of the spray as you use it. Better yet, try to avoid using it yourself.

PART TWO

Recipes for Recovery and Protection from Future Illness

Chapter 7

BEFORE YOU START COOKING

THINK OF THE ROAD TO HEALING AND REPLENISHING A depleted body as a path in the country surrounded by fields of beautiful, wholesome foods. These are the foods that are the foundation of the recipes in this book, and they are meant to help you move along that road. Each recipe has been designed to include ingredients that will, together, help optimize all of their health-enhancing and protective nutritional dividends. Most were developed to be relatively simple to prepare, and many have variations to further spark the appetite and inspire your own ideas. In addition, they are intended to be suitable, appealing, and just as beneficial for all the members of your family and anyone who wishes to consume the best kinds of foods.

The recipes have been divided into three groups that harmonize with the three phases of recovery. At the heart of the recipes are ingredients that are unaltered as much as possible by refining or processing. They aim to help meet the special needs that may arise from treatment, like the desire for sippable, mild-flavored or smooth-textured foods. These three groups are:

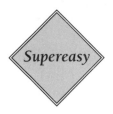

Recipes that are easy to digest and that fit well with the most demanding stages of treatment (phase one). These are sippable beverages or light meals or purees which are *Supereasy* to eat and not demanding on the digestive system.

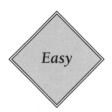

Recipes that are mild flavored, fairly soft, still relatively *Easy* to digest, but which need some ability to chew and swallow. Even though some can also be made into a puree, they were not primarily designed with pureeing in mind. These recipes are intended for that transition period during the early stages of recovery that follows the end of treatment (phase two).

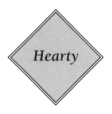

Recipes that are supernourishing and *Hearty*, requiring a normal ability to chew and swallow, an almost normal digestive system, and a normal desire to eat. Usually these will be most appealing after you have recovered from the stresses of treatment and begin to feel energetic again (phase three).

Recipe chapters are divided by types of foods and meals, and each chapter is preceded by a list of the recipes with the groupings we have just described. Each recipe is also identified by an icon. Remember, though, that any of the recipes can be enjoyed during any phase, depending on your preferences.

ABOUT THE INGREDIENTS

Whole Grains Are Central

The grain ingredients in these recipes call for whole grains. However, if your digestive tract is sensitive, you can temporarily substitute their refined counterparts, like white rice and pearled barley. Be sure the pasta you buy, though, is made from 100 percent durum wheat semolina. When you do use a refined grain, remember that you will need to shorten the cooking time from

30 to 35 minutes for brown rice to 15 to 20 minutes for white rice, and from 60 minutes for hulled barley to 30 to 45 minutes for pearled barley. Whole grain and white pasta cook in about the same amount of time. Most grains can be found in supermarkets or whole food or health food stores.

Fresh Fruits Are Emphasized

Many of the our recipes include fresh or sun-dried fruits. When unavailable, frozen, unsweetened fruits are suitable alternatives to fresh fruits, and canned fruits may also be substituted as needed. However, be aware that canned fruits can be overcooked during processing, and some nutrients can be washed away or damaged by exposure to oxygen, resulting in some loss of nutritional value. Often canned and processed fruits come with sweeteners and other added substances.

The Freshest Vegetables Are the Best

The majority of the recipes call for fresh vegetables. Special situations, such as difficulty in swallowing or digesting foods, may require special consideration of the vegetables you choose. We have primarily used those that tend to be more easily digested and that can be prepared to handle different situations, such as being left whole or prepared as a nice, smooth puree.

Sometimes during recovery, your physician or dietitian may advise you not to eat raw vegetables or unpeeled fruits that may carry microorganisms that, while totally harmless under normal conditions, may affect you when your immune system is compromised. If or when this occurs, substitute frozen or canned vegetables. For the best results, though, buy the freshest produce that is available.

If you can get vegetables from a local farmer's market, you will usually be assured of getting the freshest possible. When vegetables are out of season or unavailable, some substitutions will work well:

In a Nutshell
No matter how you feel, the primary demand of the body, second only to water, is for energy, what scientists call "calories." Calories provide energy and energy keeps us alive. Calories are one of our body's paramount needs at any time.

canned tomatoes can be used instead of fresh ones, for instance. Choose good quality, canned tomatoes—they may cost a few cents more, but you will notice the difference in flavor, appearance, and texture—all factors that are important to meal appeal—especially if you have little appetite.

Onions and garlic are liberally used   To add a dimension of flavor and texture, as well as vital compounds, garlic, onions, and related vegetables like leeks and shallots are included often in the recipes. These foods, when cooked, take on a more subtle and mellow flavor than when raw. Be sure to cook them gently, over low to moderate heat, because when fried or cooked at high temperatures, their flavors may not be pleasing. Especially take care not to burn garlic as it can take on a bitter flavor. If you desire a more bland flavored dish or want something more digestible, you can omit either the garlic, onions, or both, but expect a different flavor and, in some cases, a change in texture.

Beans, Lentils, Nuts and Seeds

Use dry beans with care   We have included only a few recipes that use whole dry cooked beans (like pintos, black beans, and kidney beans) as the primary ingredient—even though they are superstars of nutrition—because they tend to be hard to digest, particularly if the digestive tract is sensitive during or after treatment. For some persons, lima beans, black beans, and garbanzo beans seem to be among the hardest to digest, while white beans (like cannellini or small white beans) tend to be somewhat easier on the digestive system. If you desire the flavor of a bean but are concerned about its digestibility, you can remove the skin by putting them through a ricer after cooking and before adding them to the recipe. This may make the recipe smoother and thicker since the beans will no longer be whole, but they will be more easily handled by your body. When cooking your own beans is not possible, a good quality, cooked, canned bean can be used instead (see Sources, page 225). Just as with vegetables, good quality canned beans may cost a few pennies more, but you will readily see the difference in appearance, flavor, and texture.

Fresh but well-cooked beans are the best   When you choose to use the cooked dry beans called for in these recipes, you'll get the most nutrition by soaking the beans and cooking them yourself. Let's be sure, though, to thoroughly cook them since undercooked legumes (dry beans, peas, and lentils) contain some potentially toxic compounds that, when completely cooked, become harmless. Some people, though, regardless of how healthy they are, have problems with gas (flatulence) after eating beans.

Prevent gas the sure way   To minimize digestive upsets that sometimes accompany the consumption of beans, try this preparation method, which removes some of the indigestible compounds responsible for digestive upset: Put the beans in a large pot with ample water to cover. Bring the water to a boil, and keep it at a rolling boil for one minute. Turn off the heat, cover, and let soak for an hour. Then discard the soaking water, rinse the beans, and cook them in fresh water until tender.

Lentils are easy on you   One of the most easily digestible legumes are red lentils (brown and green lentils tend to be harder for the digestive tract to handle). Red lentils cook quickly (in 20 to 25 minutes) and can be simmered until they turn creamy, smooth, and golden-colored, thick soup or stew. We have included several ways to prepare lentils that will give variety and flavor to your meals, while contributing an ancient source of proteins and other nutrients. We hope you will find at least one that will be pleasing.

Tofu is a terrific addition   Tofu is a very digestible food that contains good oils and excellent protein. Made from cooked soybean milk, which has been coagulated with a calcium or magnesium salt, tofu is mild tasting and readily takes on the seasonings used in cooking. You'll find it in many forms from being an ingredient in a creamy, smooth, sippable drink to a more traditional partner in a stir fry. While tofu is found in supermarkets everywhere, your best bet for the freshest and least refined or processed versions is to buy it from an Asian market or a health food store. If you are concerned about your calcium intake, be sure and buy the tofu that is made with calcium.

Soybean milk is a great change of pace Soybean milk is a popular, high-protein substitute for those who cannot digest cow's milk. Made by grinding soybeans with water, it is available in liquid or powder form in many grocery and health food stores. It can be used as an alternative to cow's milk in any of our recipes. However, note that it contains very little calcium unless it has been added by the manufacturer, so read the label carefully. If calcium has not been added, you will need to look for other sources if soy milk is your only "milk beverage."

Miso is mightily flavorful Miso is a paste made from fermented soybeans combined with grains, usually rice and barley. It should be added at the end of cooking and dissolved into hot liquid to preserve its nutrients at their best. Miso comes in many different varieties that are often referred to by their color (e.g., red miso, brown miso, etc.) and is rich in protein and B vitamins; it also contains natural digestive enzymes and lactic acid bacteria that aid digestion. If you haven't tried it, start with a mild, light tasting one that is labeled "sweet" or "light." Some types of miso are high in sodium, so you may want to use it moderately or in place of salt. You may find miso in the supermarket, but it is most commonly found in health food stores and Asian markets.

Nuts and seeds: kernels of taste Feel free to vary the kind of nut you use in a recipe. For example, if you prefer, almonds can be used in place of walnuts. However, if you can't tolerate whole nuts or seeds at the present time, they can be omitted from any of the recipes. Don't forget about them altogether, though. Over time as you get better, you will probably find that you will be able to handle them. Start slowly—try just one piece at first, and start with almonds, pistachios, or hazelnuts. These tend to be easier on the digestive tract. Whole nuts require extensive chewing, so you may prefer to use them when you are feeling better and stronger.

Nut and seed butters are smooth foods These are the thick pastes made commonly from almonds, peanuts, and sesame seeds (called tahini). They are easier to eat than whole nuts, since they are smooth and can be thinned to desired consistency with something like applesauce. No chewing is needed. To get the most healthful variety, buy "natural" nut butters, made with just the ground nut (and salt, if you desire) rather than those that use hydrogenated fats in place of the naturally occurring good fats and/or those that have added refined sugars.

Milk, Yogurt, Cheese, and Eggs

Milk: good for just about everyone Nonfat milk is recommended primarily because of the saturated fat in regular milks. But at any time when it's difficult to eat, you may want to use a higher fat milk for extra calories. In addition, some of the recipes call for nonfat dry milk powder because it adds extra protein without added saturated fat. When you use liquid milk, buy the freshest that you can and be sure it is pasteurized. If you buy raw milk, boil it well (at a full, rolling boil for at least a minute) to kill any bacteria, as you may be especially susceptible to them when your immune system has been stressed by cancer treatments. If you cannot tolerate cow's milk, try soybean milk (see page 78) or goat's milk.

Yogurt: milk's nutritional treasure Several recipes call for yogurt, not only because yogurts are easier to digest than milk, but also because some research suggests that eating yogurt regularly may help boost your immune system due to the beneficial bacteria that it's made from. In addition, during or after treatment some people have problems, usually temporary, digesting the sugar in milk (lactose). They experience stomach cramping, bloating, and often gas. In the process of making yogurt and other related products (like kefir, which is a variety of yogurt with its own special culture), milk sugar is converted to a more easily digested substance, lactic acid. This is what gives yogurt its tangy taste. Your healthiest choice is to buy unsweetened, plain, nonfat yogurt that has no gelatins or thickeners added to it, and that was made with live, bacterial cultures. You can make your own yogurt, and in the References section (page 229) you'll find books with good recipes for yogurt making. Unusual yogurt cultures can be found in the Sources section (page 225).

Yogurt Cheese: making it is a breeze   This is another delicious way to eat yogurt, and the creamy, smooth texture and flavor of yogurt cheese readily lend it to either sweet or savory seasonings. Although not available commercially, it practically makes itself, after you fix it up to drain overnight—and we bet you'll find the few minutes of effort well worth the result (see recipe, page 210). In fact, you are the boss in this venture and can make it as thick or creamy as you prefer, depending on how long it sits. Here again the best kind of yogurt to use is one without added gelatins or thickeners, and one that contains live bacterial cultures.

Cheese, but only in small amounts   Very little cheese is used in these recipes. Most aged cheeses, such as cheddar, Swiss, or Monterey Jack, although a good source of many nutrients, are high in saturated fat. Additionally, for some people, these kinds of cheeses may not be easy to digest, especially when eaten later in the day. However, you will find recipes that include part skim ricotta cheese, which has some of the milk sugar left in it and

---

In a Nutshell

Yogurt is one of the best ways to consume the great proteins and calcium of milk, and it is much easier to digest and better tolerated than milk.

which is lower in fat than whole milk. If you prefer, you can use nonfat cottage cheese instead, though the smoother texture of ricotta cheese may be easier to eat.

Eggs: incredibly versatile

We have used eggs in some of the recipes, and with only a few exceptions where the yolk is absolutely necessary (like in a custard or souffle), you have the choice of using two egg whites for each whole egg called for. Be sure to buy the freshest eggs that you can. They have a thick white that won't run all over the pan when you cook it, and you just might notice a better flavor. Farmer's markets are often a good place to find very fresh eggs, in addition to fruits and vegetables.

Seasonings

Salt: the choice is left to you   If you are on a salt or sodium restricted diet, you can omit or limit the salt in these recipes, but recognize that the resulting salt-free or low salt dishes will have a much more mild flavor. In place of salt, you may wish to use pepper, lemon, vinegar, or other seasonings that add flavor. Some condiments like miso, tamari, and soy sauces, are also high in sodium, and a small amount may be used in place of salt to bring out flavors.

Herbs and spices for flavor and aroma   Herbs and spices such as oregano and basil and cinnamon and nutmeg are used frequently in these recipes. For the most part, dried herbs are called for since they are usually what we have in our pantries. Fresh herbs are best, of course, and if you grow your own or have access to fresh ones, use them, and use them liberally and often. Generally speaking, use one-and-a-half to twice the amount of fresh herbs when using them in place of dried ones. Fresh herbs work best when added toward the end of cooking rather than at the beginning like dried herbs.

Sweeteners and flavorings to tantalize the taste buds　Only unrefined sweeteners and pure flavorings have been used in the recipes. For example, we call for 100 percent pure maple syrup, which is the sweetest and, of course, tastes like real maple. Honey comes with its own flavor and though not significant in the small amounts we usually use, it adds a bit of healthful goodness to our food.

In a Nutshell

If you have noticed that you've become sensitive to certain flavors (there is often an enhanced sensitivity to sweetness with chemotherapy), take that into account when preparing a recipe. You may cut back on the seasonings by half to start with as you are cooking. You can always add more—much easier than having used too much in the first place.

Oils: pass the good fats, please　Primarily, oil is used as a flavor enhancer and a seasoning in our recipes. We use only small amounts, mostly to soften onions and garlic while they are cooking. Use only low to moderate heat when cooking with oil to help keep it from being damaged. Also, choose extra virgin olive oil since it is made from high quality olives and is processed without any solvents or chemicals. Olive oils can have distinctive flavors, aromas, and colors. Ask your grocer or olive oil purveyor (see Sources, page 225).

ABOUT NUTRITIONAL ANALYSIS DATA

A per-serving, nutritional breakdown is given for each recipe, based on the Food Processor nutrition analysis program. Amounts have been rounded to the nearest whole number.

Nutrient content may vary depending on specific ingredients and brands of products used. It is important, therefore, to use the analyses as only general guidlines, as both different products and different analytical programs can yield different results.

Chapter 8

SUPER SIPPABLES

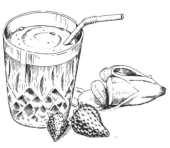

SOMETIMES WHEN YOU'RE FEELING FATIGUED AND NOT very well, smooth, sippable, high-energy and high-protein liquids may be most suitable and appealing. A Super Sippable can be a meal in itself and give you vital energy and health-enhancing substances at a time when eating solid food is not possible or appealing.

A few tips for getting the most out of your Super Sippables:

• To help prevent the blender from stalling, put liquid and soft foods into it first and then add solid pieces of foods (like fruit chunks) and ice when called for.

• If you want to boost the protein content, blend in one-third of a cup nonfat dry milk powder to your beverage, adding more liquid if the beverage becomes too thick (this is equal to the amount of protein in one cup of liquid milk).

• If you are on a low microbial diet (that provides foods with a low bacterial count to help minimize the risk of infection through the digestive tract) because your immune system is temporarily compromised, use only thick-skinned, unblemished fresh fruits that require peeling or canned, frozen, or well-cooked fresh fruits and vegetables.

• Use your imagination, be creative, and include a wide variety of colorful fruits and vegetables in your Super Sippables—not only to help stimulate your appetite and for taste, but to provide for the best possible nutrition and protection from future illness.

Super Sippables

Supereasy recipes are smooth sippable foods for ease in swallowing without need to chew.

Easy recipes are soft and tender, need some chewing but are gentle on the digestive tract.

Hearty recipes are most suitable when you are feeling well and back to normal.

Recipe	Supereasy	Easy	Hearty
Hi-Protein Pineapple Dream *(page 85)*	◆		
Juice Cubies *(page 86)*	◆		
Cool Caribbean Breeze *(page 87)*	◆		
Apricot-Mango Frozen Yogurt Smoothie *(page 88)*	◆		
Fruited Yogurt Smoothie *(page 89)*	◆		
Almond Milk *(page 90)*	◆		
Hi-Energy Soy Milk Cocoa *(page 91)*	◆		
Raspberry Kefir Smoothie *(page 92)*	◆		
Orange Refresher *(page 93)*	◆		
Peachy Lemon Smoothie *(page 94)*	◆		
Soothing Ginger Tea *(page 95)*	◆		
Veggies of the Liquid Persuasion *(page 96)*	◆		

Hi-Protein Pineapple Dream

Bonnie Bruce

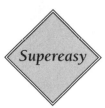

Supereasy

SERVES 2

When you want something that's high in calories and protein, yet smooth and Supereasy to eat, this will fit the bill. By varying the fruit, you can also make it easier to digest by lowering the fiber content. For example, for less fiber, use a peeled, ripe peach instead of pineapple. Also try oranges, bananas, nectarines, or apricots.

½ cup cold nonfat or 1% milk
1 cup soft tofu, drained and mashed
1¼ cups diced fresh pineapple
1 teaspoon vanilla
½ tablespoon mild honey
3 to 4 ice cubes

Put all ingredients into blender. Begin at low speed and blend until ice cubes are chopped and mixture is smooth. For a thinner drink, add more milk.

PER SERVING*
Calories: 203
Dietary fiber:
3 grams
Protein: 13 grams
Carbohydrates:
22 grams
Good fats: 5 grams
Other fats: 2 grams

With nonfat milk.

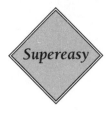

**MAKES 1
ICE CUBE TRAY**

Juice Cubies

Bonnie Bruce

These frozen chunks are extremely simple to prepare and eat. Made with fresh and natural fruit juices, you'll get all the nutritional goodness with little effort. Any kind of pure, unsweetened fruit juice will work, so use any combination that appeals to you. Possible juices you could use include: unsweetened grape juice, fresh-squeezed orange juice, orange-pineapple juice, kiwi-strawberry juice, papaya-pineapple juice, etc. As an alternative to "chunks," you can also crush the cubies into even-easier-to-eat ice chips and just let them melt in your mouth.

1 empty ice cube tray (with cube dividers)

Enough unsweetened fruit juice (fresh-squeezed when possible) to fill the ice cube tray about ⅔ full

PER JUICE
CUBIE*
*Calories: 16
Dietary fiber:
<1 gram
Protein: <1 gram
Carbohydrates:
4 grams
Good fats: <1 gram
Other fats: <1 gram*

*Made with grape juice, based on 2 tablespoons juice per cube. Nutrient values very approximate as it will depend on kind of juice used.

Pour juice into ice cube tray and freeze until solid. Remove the frozen cubes and store them in the freezer in a plastic container. Can be used one or more at a time.

To crush: Use a commercial ice crusher or crush the cubes by hand by placing 1 to 2 cubes into a heavy plastic bag and then hitting ice gently with a hammer to desired size.

VARIATION

Use the juice cubies, either crushed or whole, to chill your glasses of juice instead of regular ice cubes.

Cool Caribbean Breeze

Bonnie Bruce

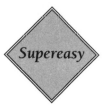

This colorful, hi-protein beverage is the essence of the tropics. Rich in vital protective substances, its mild and refreshing flavors are just right for any time of the day for either a quick pick-me-up or a light meal. Freeze the banana first if you want a thick, creamy shake.

SERVES 1 TO 2

½ cup nonfat or 1% fat milk
½ cup plain nonfat or lowfat yogurt without gelatin or
    thickeners
l large ripe banana, peeled and frozen
½ cup fresh papaya chunks
2 teaspoons pure vanilla extract
3 to 4 ice cubes

Put all ingredients into blender. Whirl until mixture is smooth. Add more yogurt for a thicker "breeze" or more milk if you'd like a thinner drink.

VARIATION

Try different varieties of fruit, such as fresh oranges and mangos instead of papaya.

PER ½ RECIPE*
Calories: 248
Dietary fiber:
4 grams
Protein: 13 grams
Carbohydrates:
49 grams
Good fats: <1 gram
Other fats: <1 gram

*Made with nonfat yogurt and nonfat milk.

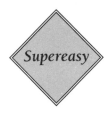

Supereasy

Apricot-Mango Frozen Yogurt Smoothie

Rowena Hubbard

SERVES 1 TO 2

Thick, cool, and delicious as a hi-energy and hi-protein breakfast drink or as a quick pick-me-up, the apricot and mango flavors give a wonderful tart-sweet taste to this smoothie. Try any flavor of yogurt that appeals to you. I buy the individual yogurt cups in my favorite flavors and put them in the freezer. That way I always have the makings of a terrific smoothie on hand.

> 1 cup (an 8-ounce carton) nonfat or lowfat apricot-mango
>   yogurt without gelatin or thickeners, frozen in its own carton
> 1 cup apricot nectar

Place frozen yogurt carton, with its top still on, under hot water and turn for a minute to loosen yogurt from carton. Empty contents into blender with the apricot nectar. Whirl until smooth.

VARIATION

PER ½ RECIPE*
Calories: 176
Dietary fiber:
<1 gram
Protein: 6 grams
Carbohydrates:
38 grams
Good fats: <1 gram
Other fats: <1 gram
_____
**Made with nonfat
yogurt and nonfat
milk.*

Try frozen peach yogurt with peach nectar, frozen strawberry yogurt with fresh orange juice, or frozen blueberry yogurt with fresh apple juice.

Fruited Yogurt Smoothie

Rowena Hubbard

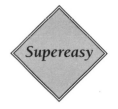

Light and easy to make, this smoothie has an excellent fruit flavor. If you want a really cold smoothie, add an ice cube to the blender mixture. I don't add honey, but you could add a teaspoon or two if you prefer a sweeter flavor.

SERVES 1 TO 2

    1 cup plain nonfat or lowfat yogurt without gelatin or
       thickeners
    ½ large ripe banana
    ½ cup fresh squeezed orange juice
    Honey or pure maple syrup to taste (optional)

Combine yogurt, banana, and juice in blender. Whirl until smooth. Stir in honey or maple syrup to taste.

VARIATION

In place of the banana, use ½ cup fresh berries, papaya chunks, mango chunks, fresh peach slices, plum slices, nectarine slices, or cantaloupe chunks, and in place of the fresh orange juice, use any favorite fresh juice.

PER ½ RECIPE*
Calories: 124
Dietary fiber:
<1 gram
Protein: 8 grams
Carbohydrates:
23 grams
Good fats: <1 gram
Other fats: <1 gram

*Made with nonfat yogurt.

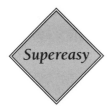

Supereasy

MAKES ABOUT
1 CUP

Almond Milk

Rowena Hubbard

Almond milk is basically a drink prepared from nuts. Other nuts such as hazelnuts can be used, and all nut milks can be drunk plain or sweetened with honey. Nut milks are especially valuable contributors of the protective nutrients and good fats, and they can be used as a change from cow's or goat's milk.

Cheesecloth

1 cup whole almonds, natural or blanched
3 or 4 ice cubes

1. Place almonds in the bowl of a food processor with metal blade in place. Place ice cubes into 2-cup glass measure and add cold water to make 1¼ cups.

2. Add iced water to almonds and process until almonds are finely crushed and ice cubes are disintegrated.

3. Place a double thickness of cheesecloth into a 2-cup strainer that has been placed over a 2-cup glass measure. Pour mixture into cheesecloth and allow to drip through. Pull ends of cheesecloth together and squeeze mixture until all moisture has drained out. Store covered in refrigerator for up to a week and a half.

PER SERVING*
Calories: 450
Dietary fiber:
8 grams
Protein: 15 grams
Carbohydrates:
16 grams
Good fats: 32 grams
Other fats: 4 grams

**Nutrient values
are very
approximate, as fat
depends on
processing and how
much pulp is left.*

Hi-Energy Soy Milk Cocoa

Rowena Hubbard

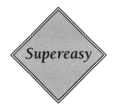

SERVES 2

You can pop this easy cocoa in the microwave to heat or make it in a saucepan on the stove. It's warming, rich tasting, and goes down easily. If there is some left over, simply cover and refrigerate. Note that cocoa contains some caffeine and related compounds. If you prefer to avoid them, replace the cocoa with unsweetened carob powder.

  1 tablespoon unsweetened dry cocoa powder
  1 to 2 tablespoons honey
  2 teaspoons pure vanilla extract
  2 cups plain soy milk

Whisk together the cocoa, honey, and vanilla in a 4-cup glass measure or a small saucepan until well mixed. Stir in soy milk.

TO MICROWAVE

Microwave ingredients in glass measure, uncovered, on high for about 3 minutes until hot. Transfer ingredients to a saucepan and warm over medium heat for 4 to 5 minutes or until foamy.

PER SERVING
Calories: 125
Dietary fiber:
4 grams
Protein: 8 grams
Carbohydrates:
17 grams
Good fats: 3 grams
Other fats: <1 gram

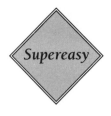

Supereasy

SERVES 1 TO 2

Raspberry Kefir Smoothie

Rowena Hubbard

Kefir is liquid yogurt and comes in many flavors, so experiment and try the variations. This, cold, thick smoothie made with kefir tastes like a rich milkshake, but it's better. Filled with high-quality protein and a great, fresh fruit taste, it also contains beneficial active yogurt-type cultures. The only thing you might find bothersome are the berry seeds; you can strain them out before serving, if you prefer.

1 cup lowfat raspberry kefir
1 cup fresh raspberries (unsweetened frozen berries may be
   substituted)
½ cup unsweetened apple juice
1 to 2 teaspoons honey (optional)

Combine all ingredients in a blender jar. Cover and whirl until smooth.

VARIATION

Try strawberry kefir with fresh strawberries or plain kefir with frozen banana slices.

PER ½ RECIPE
Calories: 105
Dietary fiber:
3 grams
Protein: 5 grams
Carbohydrates:
19 grams
Good fats: 1 gram
Other fats: 1 gram

Orange Refresher

Rowena Hubbard

This is a cool and refreshing beverage that packs a big nutrition punch with the high quality protein of soy milk. Fresh orange juice gives it the flavor of the orchard. For extra flavor and fiber, be sure to scrape the fine pulp that clings to the juicer into the glass.

½ cup plain soy milk, cold
1 cup fresh squeezed orange juice

Stir soy milk and orange juice together in a large glass.

VARIATION

Experiment with the many different fresh and natural juices that are in the supermarket.

PER SERVING
Calories: 150
Dietary fiber:
2 grams
Protein: 5 grams
Carbohydrates:
28 grams
Good fats: 2 grams
Other fats: <1 gram

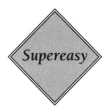

Supereasy

SERVES 1 TO 2

Peachy Lemon Smoothie

Rowena Hubbard

*Creamy, thick, and frosty, this tart smoothie has a distinct lemon fla-
vor. The natural, wholesome yogurt makes it taste so rich, you'll think
that it is made with ice cream. If lemon is too tart for you, replace half
of the lemon yogurt with vanilla yogurt, and the flavors will be softer
and peachier. I like lemon yogurt with frozen blueberries, too. Freeze
your own fruit when they are at their peak of flavor in season.*

> 1 cup (an 8-ounce carton) nonfat or lowfat lemon yogurt
>   without added gelatin or thickeners
> 1 cup fresh peach slices (unsweetened frozen peach slices may
>   be used)
> ½ cup fresh squeezed orange juice

Place all ingredients into a blender jar. Whirl until smooth.

VARIATION

Try strawberry yogurt with fresh or frozen strawberries, peach
yogurt with fresh or frozen peaches, lemon yogurt with fresh or
frozen blueberries, vanilla yogurt with any fresh or frozen fruit,
or raspberry yogurt with fresh or frozen raspberries.

PER ½ RECIPE*
*Calories: 176
Dietary fiber:
2 grams
Protein: 7 grams
Carbohydrates:
37 grams
Good fats: <1 gram
Other fats: <1 gram*

**Made with nonfat
yogurt.*

Soothing Ginger Tea

Bonnie Bruce

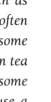

This is a nice, soothing beverage. Make it with black teas such as English Breakfast, Assam, Darjeeling, Ceylon, and what is often called "orange pekoe" on tea bags. These kinds of teas contain some antioxidants. Loose teas are usually of higher quality than teas in tea bags. Note that orange pekoe tea and other black teas contain some caffeine and related compounds. If you prefer to avoid them, use a decaffeinated tea.

1 tea bag of good quality black tea or 1 to 2 teaspoons
   loose tea
½ teaspoon chopped fresh ginger
1 (½-inch) slice of fresh orange, studded with 2 cloves
Mild flavored honey to taste

1. Bring some water to a boil.
2. Put the tea bag or loose tea leaves, fresh ginger, and orange slice into a 2-cup measure or small tea pot that has been rinsed with hot water.
3. Add boiling water to the cup and let steep for 2 to 3 minutes.
4. Strain hot tea into cup and sweeten with honey as desired.

VARIATION

Try other flavored or herbal teas that, combined with the flavor of ginger, are appealing to you.

PER SERVING*
Calories: 16
Dietary fiber:
<1 gram
Protein: <1 gram
Carbohydrates:
4 grams
Good fats: <1 gram
Other fats: <1 gram
_____
*Before adding honey.

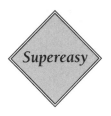

Supereasy

SERVINGS VARY

Veggies of the Liquid Persuasion

Gene Spiller

A vegetable juice is a super choice as a treasure chest of protective, easy-to-digest phytochemicals, after you have satisfied your need for calories and protein. Try to use carrots and some dark green leaves and celery as much as you can for their richness in nutrition. Vegetable juices are something you should drink when you feel the need for concentrated nutrition. Hundreds of combinations can be created. You can make simple juices from a single vegetable or you can make multi-veggie juices that combine many vegetables.

About vegetable juicers Some juicing machines remove the fiber, others do not. Both kinds of machines have a place in the kitchen. To make a fiber-free juice, you need a good juicer that separates the pulp from the liquid with enough power so that only the fiber and little else is left behind (see Shopping Sources, page 225). To make a juice with fiber, use a powerful blender or one of the special machines that have the extra power to make your vegetable into a true juice-like beverage. These machines last a lifetime, so investing in one is worthwhile.

Two types of juices Vegetable juices without the fiber are clear liquids that are very easy to drink. This type of juice is almost a "supplement" of phytochemicals. Juices with the pulp in are liquid foods with the advantages of fiber but are as easy to drink in large quantities.

Which is better? Both types are good, as they help to enrich your diet in different ways. In the case of vegetables like broccoli or cabbage that are loaded with a good protection but that appear hard to digest during treatment, preparing them in a juicer that removes the fiber is a good way to add them to your diet. Remember that if the fiber is gone, you should get your fiber somewhere else.

Preparing your vegetables   Clean vegetables well. Wash green leaves, and wash and scrub vegetables like carrots or celery. Follow any additional directions given by the manufacturer of your machine.

Single vegetable juices   Carrot, celery, and tomatoes make excellent juices, but try any vegetable recommended by the manufacturer that sounds appealing.

Multi-veggie juices   Mixed juices give you a wider range of phytochemicals and flavors. The number of combinations is endless. The following recipes are just a few examples—use the guidelines from the manufacturer of your machine to prepare these juices.

Carrot-Celery Delight

3 to 6 carrots (depending on size)
2 to 3 celery stalks
⅓ cucumber, peeled
1 ripe, medium-size tomato

Carrot-Buttermilk Blend

3 to 6 carrots (depending on size)
1 ripe, medium-size tomato
½ cup buttermilk

Spinach-Tomato Blend

10 to 15 leaves fresh spinach
2 to 3 ripe, medium-size tomatoes
1 celery stalk
1 medium carrot

Carrot Juice with Apples or Peaches

3 to 6 carrots (depending on size)
2 to 4 cored apples or seeded peaches

VARIATION

For added calories and protein, add some buttermilk or yogurt to the juices. Also, sun-dried raisins can be added to blender-type juices.

PER SERVING
Nutritional value will vary widely, depending on the kinds and quantity of vegetables.

Chapter 9

ELEGANT EGGS

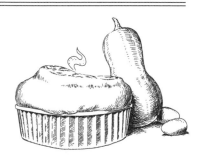

AN IDEAL SOURCE OF PROTEIN TO HELP THE BODY HEAL
and rebuild, the nourishing elegant egg has been at the center of bat-
tle primarily because of its cholesterol content and its potential con-
tribution to heart disease. At last, though, we have finally learned
that the egg doesn't deserve such a shadowy reputation. In cancer,
and in heart disease, it is clearly saturated fat that is the bigger cul-
prit. This is especially good news for the cancer survivor. However
you're feeling, a cooked egg will give you some energy and is an
excellent source of a nearly perfect protein. Tips for eggs:

• Don't eat them raw or blend raw eggs into beverages—there's
too big a risk of bacterial contamination (even if you aren't sick); it's
also a good idea to refrain from eating undercooked, soft cooked, or
sunny-side-up eggs where the egg white isn't thoroughly cooked,
especially if your immune system is low.

• If you are concerned about the cholesterol in eggs, substitute
two egg whites (which are almost pure protein) for each egg called
for. There is no cholesterol in the white. However, this substitution
won't work in souffles or many custards.

• To add some easily digested egg protein to foods, hard cook
the egg, chop it, and then sprinkle it over cooked vegetables, like
spinach or other leafy greens.

Elegant Eggs

Supereasy recipes are smooth sippable foods for ease in swallowing without need to chew.

Easy recipes are soft and tender, need some chewing but are gentle on the digestive tract.

Hearty recipes are most suitable when you are feeling well and back to normal.

Recipe	Supereasy	Easy	Hearty
Incredible Versatile Eggs *(page 101)*		◆	
Winter Squash Soufflé *(page 103)*		◆	
Baked Honey-Yogurt Custard *(page 104)*		◆	
Orange-Tofu Custard *(page 105)*		◆	
Hi-Protein Egg Patties *(page 106)*		◆	
Banana-Walnut Custard *(page 107)*		◆	◆

Incredible Versatile Eggs

Bonnie Bruce

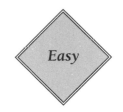

SERVES 2

One of the easiest foods to digest and one of the best for nourishment and healing, eggs combine very well with the plant sources of phytochemicals. Eggs can be eaten in an almost endless number of ways by varying the ingredients and preparing them slightly differently. Here are a few ideas to inspire you.

Basic Eggs

1 tablespoon extra virgin olive oil
2 large whole eggs
1 large egg white
Salt and freshly ground pepper to taste

1. Gently warm 1 to 2 tablespoons of water with the olive oil in a skillet (do not overheat).
2. Beat the eggs in a bowl. Add herbs as suggested below or leave plain.
3. Pour the eggs into the pan. Stir gently while eggs are cooking to prevent sticking. Cook to desired consistency. Serve on a toasted piece of whole grain bread and top with a few slices of ripe avocado and/or tomato. Salt and pepper to taste.

Egg Frittata

Increase number of whole eggs to 4. Before cooking eggs, cook about 1 cup shredded white potatoes or red garnet yams in a small amount of olive oil until tender. Stir ½ teaspoon dried basil leaves into the eggs before adding them to the cooked potatoes. Cook egg and potato mixture in the olive oil–water mixture over low to moderate heat until eggs are set. Add salt and pepper to taste. Serve topped with chopped fresh tomatoes and Italian parsley.

(continues)

Spinach or Sorrel Omelet

Increase number of whole eggs to 4. Combine 1 cup cooked, drained, and chopped fresh spinach or sorrel leaves and ½ teaspoon dried tarragon leaves with eggs. Cook gently in the olive oil–water mixture until eggs are cooked to desired doneness. Add salt and pepper to taste. Top with a dollop of yogurt and chopped fresh chives.

Egg and Yogurt Scramble

Increase number of whole eggs to 4. Stir ¼ cup plain nonfat or lowfat yogurt and 1 tablespoon each finely chopped fresh parsley, chives, and basil into eggs. Cook gently in olive oil–water mixture until eggs are cooked to desired doneness. Add salt and pepper to taste. Complement this slightly tart scramble by topping it with orange marmalade or a jam of your choice.

PER SERVING*
Calories: 122
Dietary fiber:
<1 gram
Protein: 8 grams
Carbohydrates:
<1 gram
Good fats: 8 grams
Other fats: 2 grams
———
*For Basic Eggs.

Winter Squash Soufflé

Bonnie Bruce

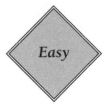

This is the easiest soufflé recipe I have ever made. It rises high and light, and has a wonderful, mildly sweet flavor and an appealing light golden color. Easy to digest, it is a recipe that contains an abundance of good protein and protective nutrients.

SERVES 4

2½ pounds (4 to 5 cups) cooked and mashed butternut or
    kabocha squash
2 tablespoons pure maple syrup
⅛ teaspoon freshly grated nutmeg
½ teaspoon salt (optional)
4 large whole eggs, separated

1. Preheat oven to 350 degrees. Lightly oil a 2-quart soufflé or casserole dish.

2. Thoroughly mix the cooked squash, maple syrup, nutmeg, salt (if using), and egg yolks in a blender or food processor until smooth. (If you use a blender, you may have to add the squash in two or three batches and scrape the sides down).

3. Beat egg whites until stiff in a large bowl and gently fold the squash mixture into the beaten egg whites.

4. Turn mixture into the baking dish. Bake 40 to 45 minutes or until soufflé is puffed, brown, and set. Serve with bright green wilted or steamed fresh spinach leaves for a colorful and absolutely delicious light meal.

PER SERVING
Calories: 209
Dietary fiber:
7 grams
Protein: 8 grams
Carbohydrates:
33 grams
Good fats: 3 grams
Other fats: 2 grams

VARIATION

Substitute other winter squash, like banana or Danish, for the butternut or kabocha squash.

Baked Honey-Yogurt Custard

Rowena Hubbard

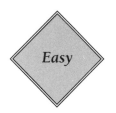

Easy

SERVES 2

Rich tasting but a little tart, this golden custard is smooth and flavorful. I find that putting the custard cups into a loaf pan allows the water to come almost to the tops of the custard cups. This keeps the mixture cooking at an even temperature and prevents separation.

1 cup plain nonfat or lowfat yogurt without gelatin and
    thickeners
2 large whole eggs
3 to 4 tablespoons honey
2 teaspoons pure vanilla extract
Pinch of freshly grated nutmeg

1. Preheat oven to 350 degrees. Whisk together yogurt and eggs in a large bowl until very well mixed. Blend in honey, vanilla, and a pinch of nutmeg.

2. Pour into two ceramic custard cups (holding ¾ cup each—if using glass cups you may need three of them). Place in a deep pan and fill pan with hot tap water to reach almost to the top of the custard cups.

3. Bake for 30 minutes or until a knife inserted into the center comes out clean. Remove cups from water and cool. Cover and chill until ready to serve.

PER SERVING*
Calories: 269
Dietary fiber:
1 gram
Protein: 14 grams
Carbohydrates:
42 grams
Good fats: 3 grams
Other fats: 2 grams

*Made with nonfat
yogurt.*

VARIATION

Substitute pure maple syrup for the honey for a different flavor.

Orange-Tofu Custard

Rowena Hubbard

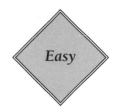

Easy

Not quite as creamy as custard made with milk, the tofu custard does have a smooth texture and high quality protein. Be sure not to over-cook this custard or it will separate.

1 cup soft tofu, crumbled
2 large egg yolks
2 tablespoons honey
½ teaspoon fresh grated orange peel
1 teaspoon arrowroot
1 teaspoon pure vanilla extract
Pinch of freshly grated nutmeg

1. Preheat oven to 300 degrees. Whisk together soft tofu and egg yolks until well blended. Then add honey, orange peel, arrow-root, vanilla, and nutmeg, and mix until mixture is smooth.

2. Pour into two ceramic custard cups (holding ¾ cup each—if using glass cups you may need three of them). Place in a deep pan and fill pan with hot tap water to reach almost to the top of custard cups.

3. Bake for 25 to 30 minutes or until a knife inserted in the center comes out clean. Remove cups from water and cool. Cover and chill until ready to serve.

PER SERVING
Calories: 213
Dietary fiber:
2 grams
Protein: 13 grams
Carbohydrates:
20 grams
Good fats: 2 grams
Other fats: 7 grams

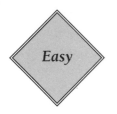

Easy

SERVES 4

Hi-Protein Egg Patties

Bonnie Bruce

The combination of the good quality plant protein in tofu with the excellent protein in eggs gives this easy-to-digest recipe a protein wallop. These patties are good served as a light entree or as a sandwich filler on a whole grain bun. They can be varied by substituting basil or adding garlic, or using other herbs that you fancy, instead of the oregano.

1 cup soft tofu, mashed
¼ cup plain nonfat or lowfat yogurt without gelatin and
   thickeners
2 large whole eggs, slightly beaten
1 cup raw wheat germ
½ to 1 teaspoon dried oregano leaves
Salt and freshly ground pepper to taste

1. Preheat oven to 375 degrees. Mix the mashed tofu, yogurt, eggs, wheat germ, and oregano together until well combined.

2. Shape into four patties about ½" to ¾" thick. Place onto nonstick or lightly oiled baking sheet.

3. Bake for 25 to 30 minutes, or until browned and firm to the touch. Season to taste with salt and pepper. Serve with your favorite side dishes and condiments. Apricot jam or a spicy fruit chutney (like mango) goes very well with these patties.

PER SERVING*
Calories: 196
Dietary fiber:
4 grams
Protein: 15 grams
Carbohydrates:
16 grams
Good fats: 6 grams
Other fats: 2 grams

―――――
**Made with nonfat
yogurt.*

Banana-Walnut Custard

Bonnie Bruce

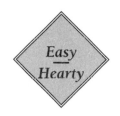

Delicious either warm or chilled, this custard is rich and sweet fla-vored with the crunch of walnuts. It's a great hi-energy food for breakfast, dessert, or as a snack. If you would prefer the smooth, creamy texture of custard simply with the tenderness and mild flavor of banana, the walnuts can be omitted.

SERVES 6

2 ripe, medium-size bananas
½ cup chopped walnuts
¼ cup freshly squeezed orange juice
1 tablespoon tapioca
2 large whole eggs
4 to 5 tablespoons honey
1 tablespoon pure vanilla extract
1½ cups part skim ricotta cheese
½ cup plain nonfat or lowfat yogurt without gelatin or
    thickeners
1 teaspoon grated fresh lemon peel

1. Preheat oven to 350 degrees. Lightly oil a 9-inch round or square baking dish. Make one layer of ¼-inch banana slices over bottom of the dish. Sprinkle with the chopped walnuts, if using.

2. Put remaining ingredients into blender or food processor, and mix until smooth. Pour into the baking dish over the bananas and walnuts.

3. Bake for 40 to 45 minutes or until edges are brown and a knife inserted into the center comes out clean. Let cool for 10 minutes before serving.

VARIATION

Add a yogurt "frosting" by combining 2 tablespoons honey with 1 cup yogurt and spreading over the top of the custard after it has cooled.

PER SERVING*
Calories: 249
Dietary fiber:
1 gram
Protein: 12 grams
Carbohydrates:
30 grams
Good fats: 5 grams
Other fats: 4 grams

Made with
walnuts and nonfat
yogurt.

Chapter 10

STELLAR SOUPS

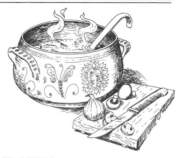

NOURISHING, WARMING, AND FILLING, SOUPS HAVE BEEN served as the main course or to complement meals for millennia. Good soups begin with good, wholesome ingredients. This section contains a wide variety of soups, all made with fresh, unrefined foods. They range from very light, Supereasy to swallow and digest, creamy-textured purees to Hearty soups full of texture and flavor. All are a valuable source of energy and contain a range of vitamins, minerals, and protective compounds. We have included ideas for variations so that you can make an easy or hearty recipe easier to eat, if you wish.

Herbs and spices are essential ingredients in these soups because they give both flavor and health-giving properties. For example, parsley adds a mild, delicate flavor and is high in vitamin C, one of the precious antioxidant vitamins. Garlic and onions have long been celebrated for their salubrious properties, such as helping to prevent infections; and some research has shown that garlic and onions contain phytochemicals that help prevent certain types of cancer. Here are a few soup-making tips:

• Make a large batch of the Simple Vegetable Stock (page 207) and keep it frozen. Many of the recipes call for water or vegetable stock. Using the stock adds to the soup's flavor quality in addition to contributing vital nutrients.

• Taste your soup before salting it. The fresh flavors of the ingredients may be perfect as is.

• We cook the onions and garlic (when called for) first because it softens and sweetens their flavors. If you'd like to omit that step, you can simply add garlic and onions to the mixture during simmering. If you prefer a milder soup, they can be omitted.

Stellar Soups

Supereasy recipes are smooth sippable foods for ease in swallowing without need to chew.

Easy recipes are soft and tender, need some chewing but are gentle on the digestive tract.

Hearty recipes are most suitable when you are feeling well and back to normal.

Recipe	*Supereasy*	*Easy*	*Hearty*
Creamy Potato and Yam Soup *(page 111)*	◆		
Puree of Fresh Fennel *(page 112)*	◆		
Astounding Avocado Soup *(page 113)*	◆		
Harvest Squash and Apple Soup *(page 114)*	◆		
Dilled Carrot and Yam Soup *(page 116)*	◆		
Broccoli Bisque *(page 117)*	◆		
Simply Miso *(page 118)*	◆		
Miso Soup with Sticky Rice *(page 119)*	◆	◆	
Miso Soup with Spinach and Yams *(page 120)*		◆	
Pasta in Brodo di Casa *(page 121)*		◆	
Potato Soup with Spinach Ribbons *(page 122)*		◆	
Golden Red Lentil Soup *(page 123)*	◆	◆	
Pasta and Mushroom Chowder *(page 124)*		◆	
Red Lentil Soup with Fresh Greens *(page 125)*		◆	
Ziti and Cannellini Hot Pot *(page 126)*		◆	◆
Barley and Friends *(page 128)*		◆	
Mediterranean Minestrone Pronto *(page 128)*			◆
Hearty Green Lentil Soup Provençal *(page 130)*			◆
Miso Soup with Buckwheat Noodles and Beans *(page 132)*			◆

Creamy Potato and Yam Soup

Bonnie Bruce

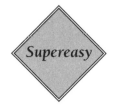

SERVES 4

Fortified by nature's bounty, this smooth and thick, golden-colored soup is delicious warm or cold. It has a mild, slightly rich flavor from the red garnet yams which is tempered by the slight tanginess of the yogurt. You can make this soup very thick or add milk to thin.

1 tablespoon extra virgin olive oil
1 large onion, chopped
2 medium boiling potatoes, peeled and sliced thin
2 medium red garnet yams, peeled and sliced thin
2 cups water or Simple Vegetable Stock (page 207)
¼ to ½ cup nonfat or 1% lowfat milk
¼ cup dry nonfat milk powder
¼ cup fresh chopped chives, or 2 tablespoons dried chives
1 cup plain nonfat or lowfat yogurt without gelatin or
   thickeners
Salt and freshly ground pepper

1. Gently warm the oil in a large soup kettle. Cook onion over moderate heat until tender, about 5 minutes. Add potatoes, yams, and water or stock. Cover and boil gently for 10 to 20 minutes until potatoes are tender (the yams may take a bit longer to cook than the potatoes).

2. When the onion and potatoes are soft, process or blend them with the cooking liquid to desired consistency. Return mixture to pan and add milk to desired thickness. Then stir in milk powder and chives. Reheat to desired temperature, but do not boil.

3. Let sit for a few minutes, then stir in yogurt. Season to taste with salt and pepper.

PER SERVING*
*Calories: 247
Dietary fiber:
4 grams
Protein: 9 grams
Carbohydrates:
46 grams
Good fats: 3 grams
Other fats: <1 gram*

**Made with water,
nonfat milk, and
nonfat yogurt.*

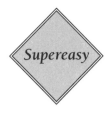

Puree of Fresh Fennel

Bonnie Bruce

Rich in carotenoids, this member of the parsley family, sometimes called anise, can be found in the produce section of most markets. It makes a delightful, mild flavored soup. This recipe gives a creamy-mouth feel from the potatoes, and it also purees well if you want something that is smooth and takes little energy to eat.

1 tablespoon extra virgin olive oil
½ medium onion, minced
3 bulbs fennel with stalks, bottom and tough outer layer removed, then quartered and cut into ¼-inch slices (about 4 cups)
2 tablespoons chopped fresh Italian parsley
2 cups water or Simple Vegetable Stock (page 207)
3 small red skinned or Yukon gold potatoes, peeled if desired, and cut into ½-inch cubes
¾ cup red garnet yam, peeled if desired, and cut into ½-inch cubes
Salt and freshly ground pepper
Yogurt (plain without gelatin or thickeners) for garnish

1. Gently warm the oil in a soup kettle. Add onion, fennel slices, and parsley. Cook over low heat until fennel is tender, about 10 to 15 minutes, stirring frequently.

2. Add water or stock, potatoes, and yam pieces. Bring to a boil. Stir and lower heat. Cook at a low boil for 20 to 25 minutes until potatoes are soft. Season to taste with salt and pepper. Serve with a dollop of yogurt on top.

VARIATION

For added protein, stir in 1/3 cup nonfat dry milk powder after potatoes are cooked. For added color, texture, flavor, and nutrients, add some diced fresh tomatoes to the soup toward the end of cooking.

PER SERVING
Calories: 126
Dietary fiber:
3 grams
Protein: 2 grams
Carbohydrates:
22 grams
Good fats: 4 grams
Other fats: <1 gram

Astounding Avocado Soup

Bonnie Bruce

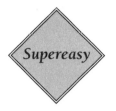

Avocado is chock full of health-enhancing and healing substances, as well as good fats. This chilled, creamy, smooth soup is quite rich and can be thinned to be straw-sippable. For added texture and color, drop in pieces of bright red, ripe, fresh diced tomatoes just before serving.

SERVES 4

1 tablespoon extra virgin olive oil
½ cup finely chopped celery stalk
2 large cloves garlic, peeled and chopped
⅓ cup finely chopped green onion
2 to 3 cups nonfat or 1% lowfat milk
1½ large ripe Haas avocados, peeled and diced
Salt and freshly ground pepper

1. Gently warm the oil. Cook celery, garlic, and onion over low to moderate heat until celery is tender and without letting the onion or garlic brown; about 10 minutes.

2. Pour one cup of milk into blender or food processor. Add cooked celery, garlic, and onion, and the avocado pieces. Begin blending at low speed and then increase blender speed as soup mixture becomes smooth. Slowly add another cup of milk and continue to blend. Check consistency and add more milk if desired. Season to taste with salt and pepper.

3. Pour into storage container and refrigerate covered until thoroughly chilled. Keep leftovers refrigerated.

PER SERVING*
Calories: 207
Dietary fiber:
3 grams
Protein: 10 grams
Carbohydrates:
17 grams
Good fats: 9 grams
Other fats: 2 grams

*Made with nonfat milk.

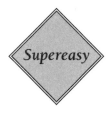

Supereasy

SERVES 2 TO 3

Harvest Squash and Apple Soup

Rowena Hubbard

Mellow in flavor with a hint of apple, this squash soup has a beautiful golden color reminiscent of a bountiful harvest. Try it with winter squashes such as kabocha, Hubbard, banana, turban, buttercup, or butternut. Making soup is a perfect way to use leftovers, so if you plan to have squash as a vegetable at one meal, cook a large one and you'll have extra for this delectable soup. Once the squash is cooked, the soup can be prepared in less than 30 minutes.

The applesauce and fresh ginger make a big difference in this recipe. Their pure flavors come through with a punch.

1 pound uncooked (about 1½ cups cooked) winter squash, cut into small chunks
1 tablespoon extra virgin olive oil
¾ cup minced onion
1 large clove garlic, peeled and minced
1 cup unsweetened applesauce
¼ to ½ teaspoon grated fresh ginger
Pinch nutmeg
Salt and freshly ground pepper
Yogurt (plain without gelatin or thickeners) and parsley for garnish

PER ½ RECIPE
Calories: 202
Dietary fiber:
7 grams
Protein: 2 grams
Carbohydrates:
35 grams
Good fats: 6 grams
Other fats: <1 gram

1. *To cook squash:* Put squash chunks and 2 to 3 cups water (depending on dryness of squash) into a large soup pan with a lid. Cover and cook until tender, about 20 to 25 minutes, depending on squash variety. Remove squash from water. Reserve the cooking water. Peel cooked squash and mash into chunks or puree to desired texture.

2. In a small skillet, gently warm the oil and cook onion over moderate heat until translucent. Stir in garlic and cook until soft, without browning.

3. Add onion-garlic mixture, applesauce, and cooked squash to the reserved cooking water in the soup pan. (If using precooked squash, add 2 to 3 cups fresh water to the pan at this time.) Stir in ginger and nutmeg.

4. Bring soup to a boil, turn heat down, and cover. Simmer 15 minutes to let flavors blend. Season to taste with salt and pepper. Serve topped with a dollop of yogurt and garnished with parsley.

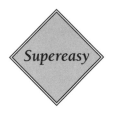

Supereasy

SERVES 6

Dilled Carrot and Yam Soup

Bonnie Bruce

Full of health-enhancing substances from nature's own pharmacy, this tummy-warming soup isn't spicy, but it's flavorful enough to pique your taste buds. It blends very nicely into a smooth, easy-to-eat light main dish or first course.

1 tablespoon extra virgin olive oil

1 medium onion, chopped

2 large cloves garlic, chopped

¼ cup slivered blanched almonds (optional)

1½ pounds carrots, scrubbed or peeled and cut into 1-inch-thick coins (4 to 5 cups)

1 medium red garnet yam, peeled and cut into 1-inch cubes (about 1½ cups)

3 cups water or Simple Vegetable Stock (page 207)

1 teaspoon dried dillweed (or 2 teaspooons chopped fresh dill)

Salt and freshly ground pepper

1 cup plain nonfat or lowfat yogurt without gelatin or thickeners

1. Gently warm the oil. Cook onion, garlic, and almonds (if using) over moderate heat until onion is tender, but not brown; about 5 to 10 minutes.

2. Add carrots, yam pieces, water or stock, and dillweed to the pan. Bring to a boil. Lower heat and boil gently for 10 to 15 minutes or until vegetables are tender. Reserve cooking liquid.

3. Put half the vegetables in a food processor or blender. Add some of the cooking liquid and puree to desired thickness. Then return to pan. Repeat with the remaining vegetables and liquid, discarding any unused liquid. Season to taste with salt and pepper. Heat very slowly and whisk in the yogurt just before serving.

PER SERVING*
Calories: 197
Dietary fiber:
5 grams
Protein: 7 grams
Carbohydrates:
31 grams
Good fats: 5 grams
Other fats: <1 gram

*Made with almonds and nonfat yogurt.

Broccoli Bisque

Bonnie Bruce

SERVES 4

This soup is mild flavored, appealingly colorful, and chock full of protective nutrients. Science has long recognized that cruciferous vegetables like broccoli contain cancer-fighting properties. This soup purees nicely into a creamy texture, making it very smooth and easy to eat.

1 tablespoon extra virgin olive oil
1 bay leaf
1 cup chopped onion
4 cups chopped fresh broccoli, including stems
2 cups water or Simple Vegetable Stock (page 207)
2 teaspoons tamari sauce
1½ cups nonfat or 1% milk
⅛ teaspoon ground allspice
½ teaspoon dried basil leaves
½ cup plain nonfat or lowfat yogurt without gelatin or thickeners
Salt and freshly ground pepper

1. Gently warm the oil with the bay leaf in a soup kettle. Add onion and cook over moderate heat until translucent. Add broccoli, water or stock, and tamari sauce. Cook covered until broccoli is tender but still bright green, about 10 minutes. Remove bay leaf.

2. In a blender, a small portion at a time, whirl a small amount of the broccoli mixture to desired consistency. Add milk to thin to desired consistency as you blend.

3. Return the soup to the pan and stir in the allspice, basil, and yogurt. Warm the soup over very low heat, so the yogurt won't curdle. Season to taste with salt and pepper.

VARIATION

Add ½ cup chopped sweet potatoes or carrots with the broccoli for more flavor and texture.

PER SERVING*
Calories: 140
Dietary fiber:
3 grams
Protein: 9 grams
Carbohydrates:
17 grams
Good fats: 3 grams
Other fats: 1 gram

Made with
vegetable stock.

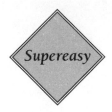

Supereasy

SERVES 1

Simply Miso

Bonnie Bruce

This is a Supereasy to eat and digest, almost instant soup that will be welcome even when you're feeling weak or run down. It has a mild flavor that's quite nourishing and soothing to the digestive tract. It's almost effortless to prepare and can be varied as you prefer. Don't let the miso boil after adding it to the soup, since boiling destroys some of the healthful substances. When its ready, just sit back and enjoy as you sip its delicious goodness.

1½ tablespoons miso (any kind)

Combine ¾ to 1 cup water and miso in a cup. Mash or stir until miso is completely dissolved. Heat in microwave for about 1½ minutes or to desired temperature.

VARIATIONS

• Stir ¼ to ½ cup diced soft tofu into water before microwaving.

• Put ½ chopped red-skinned or new potato, sweet potato (peeled if desired), or winter squash (peeled) into a cup of plain water. Microwave for about 2 minutes, until potato or squash is soft and cooked thoroughly. Stir in miso and it's ready.

• Put ½ cup scrubbed and chopped carrot into a cup of plain water. Microwave for about 2 minutes, until carrot is soft and cooked thoroughly. Stir in miso and it's ready to eat.

• Put ½ cup cauliflower, broccoli florets, or shredded cabbage into a cup of plain water and microwave until tender (about 2 to 3 minutes). Then stir in miso.

• Also try other vegetables or combinations of vegetables in the miso, such as rutabagas, turnips, parsnips, summer squash, tomatoes, fresh chopped greens, onions, garlic, etc.

PER 1-CUP
SERVING*
Calories: 49
Dietary fiber:
1 gram
Protein: 3 grams
Carbohydrates:
7 grams
Good fats: 1 gram
Other fats: <1 gram

Plain miso.

Miso Soup with Sticky Rice

Rowena Hubbard

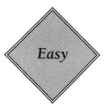

Easy

SERVES 4

This is a nourishing soup with a soothing, mild flavor that's a comfort food much like an Asian breakfast soup. Short grain rice is essential to the texture of this soup. Long grain rice simply gets mushy and doesn't produce the slightly thickened broth that makes this soup so distinctive and appealing. White short grain rice may be substituted if you'd prefer something easier to digest, but reduce cooking time to 15 to 20 minutes for white rice.

½ cup short grain brown rice, uncooked
½ teaspoon grated fresh ginger
Salt to taste
2 tablespoons light miso
¼ pound (⅓ to ⅔ cup) soft tofu, chopped
Chopped parsley for garnish

1. Combine rice, ginger, and a dash of salt with 3 cups of water in a large saucepan with a lid. Bring to boil. Cover and turn heat down. Simmer for 35 to 40 minutes or until rice is very tender.
2. Meanwhile combine miso, tofu, and 3 tablespoons water in a small bowl. Whisk together until very smooth.
3. When rice is cooked, remove from heat and swirl in miso mixture. Check seasoning and salt to taste. Serve garnished with parsley if desired.

PER SERVING
Calories: 129
Dietary fiber:
1 gram
Protein: 5 grams
Carbohydrates:
25 grams
Good fats: 1 gram
Other fats: <1 gram

Miso Soup with Spinach and Yams

Rowena Hubbard

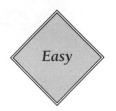

Easy

SERVES 2

"Shiro" brown miso, made from mild rice and soybean and often called Hawaiian-style, gives this soup a delicate flavor that enhances the custard-like soft tofu and doesn't overpower the vegetable flavors. Appealing with the golden orange pieces of yam and bright green shreds of spinach, this soup packs a nutrition punch. When using miso, it's easiest to blend it with a little water before adding to the dish (just swirl it into the liquid). Never boil miso. Boiling destroys the enzymes, so it's important to just stir it in at the last minute after the soup is off the heat.

½ cup red garnet yam, peeled if desired and diced to the size of small peas

¼ teaspoon grated fresh ginger

1 tablespoon soy sauce

2 cups fresh spinach leaves, chopped

4 to 6 ounces (about ⅔ cup) soft tofu, chopped or cubed

2 to 3 tablespoons shiro miso

1. Pour 2 cups water into a large microwave safe bowl. Add yam pieces, ginger, and soy sauce. Cover bowl with plastic wrap. Microwave on high 8 minutes, turning bowl after 4 minutes.

2. Remove from microwave oven and stir in spinach and tofu.

3. Blend miso with 3 tablespoons water and swirl into soup. Serve hot.

PER SERVING
Calories: 172
Dietary fiber:
5 grams
Protein: 12 grams
Carbohydrates:
22 grams
Good fats: 4 grams
Other fats: <1 gram

Pasta in Brodo di Casa

Bonnie Bruce

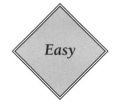

Easy

SERVES 4

Simple and quick to prepare, this version of an Italian classic is made with vegetable stock and contains the powerful impact of phytochemicals in a soothing and easy-to-eat light main dish or first course.

6 cups Simple Vegetable Stock (page 207) or mild-flavored miso
1½ cups uncooked small pasta shells (whole wheat or 100% durum semolina flour)

Bring broth to a boil. Add pasta and boil gently until pasta is cooked, about 5 to 6 minutes. Or if using miso, boil pasta in water until cooked. Then mix 2 tablespoons miso with 2 tablespoons water until well blended and stir into cooked pasta and water.

VARIATIONS

• Add diced zucchini, diced tomatoes, ¼ to ½ teaspoon dried basil leaves to boiling water and cook with pasta.
• Add finely shredded carrots, thinly sliced green onions, and ¼ teaspoon dillweed when you add the pasta.
• For added protein, add a well beaten egg or egg white during the last few minutes of cooking the pasta, stirring until egg is cooked.

PER SERVING*
Calories: 144
Dietary fiber:
1 gram
Protein: 7 grams
Carbohydrates:
29 grams
Good fats: <1 gram
Other fats: <1 gram

*Made with vegetable stock.

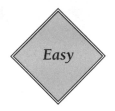

Easy

SERVES 4 TO 5

Potato Soup with Spinach Ribbons

Bonnie Bruce

When your appetite lags, it sometimes helps to "eat with your eyes." This is a colorful and delicious soup that packs a protective punch of nutrients from the carrots and spinach.

1 tablespoon extra virgin olive oil
1 medium onion, chopped
1 cup finely chopped celery stalk, including leaves
4 red skinned potatoes, peeled, if desired, and cut into ½-inch cubes
1 carrot, cut into ¼-inch coins
2 cups nonfat or 1% lowfat milk
3 cups fresh spinach leaves, washed and sliced into thin strips
Salt and freshly ground pepper
1 cup plain nonfat or lowfat yogurt without gelatin or thickeners (optional)

1. Gently warm the oil. Cook onion and celery over moderate heat until tender, stirring regularly, about 5 to 10 minutes.

2. Add potatoes, carrot, and milk. Bring to a boil, then reduce heat and simmer covered until vegetables are tender, about 20 minutes. Stir in spinach leaves and heat gently for an additional 5 minutes. Season to taste with salt and pepper. Stir in yogurt before serving.

VARIATIONS

• For more protective nutrients, add 2 chopped garlic cloves and ½ cup diced red garnet yams with the potatoes, carrot, and milk.

• If you'd like a smoother soup, the potato mixture can be pureed *before* adding the spinach. If you puree this soup with the spinach, it turns an odd shade of green.

PER ¼ RECIPE*
Calories: 223
Dietary fiber:
4 grams
Protein: 8 grams
Carbohydrates:
40 grams
Good fats: 3 grams
Other fats: <1 gram

*Made without the yogurt.

Golden Red Lentil Soup

Rowena Hubbard

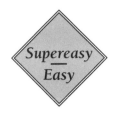

MAKES 6 TO 8
CUPS

Filled with fiber and flavor, red lentils are the fastest cooking and most easily digestible member of the lentil family. When done, they turn a lovely golden color. Cumin adds a nice subtle flavor to this simple-to-make soup, and if you would like it more robust, add another ½ teaspoon. The dollop or two of yogurt on top of the soup is essential. It adds just the right tang to perk up the finish, and adds some good protein too. Serve this soup with slices of crusty whole wheat bread.

1 tablespoon extra virgin olive oil
1 medium onion, finely chopped
1 large clove garlic, peeled and minced
1½ teaspoons ground cumin
Pinch hot chili pepper
1 cup uncooked red lentils
2 cups shredded carrots
Salt and freshly ground pepper
Plain nonfat or lowfat yogurt without gelatin or thickeners

1. Gently warm the oil in a large soup kettle. Cook onion in oil over moderate heat until just translucent. Stir in garlic and cook until lightly browned. Stir in cumin and chili pepper and cook 1 minute more to develop flavor.

2. Stir in lentils, carrots, and 4 cups of water. Bring to a boil, cover, and simmer 20 to 25 minutes until lentils are cooked and carrots are tender. Check the soup after 10 minutes and add more water if it gets too thick. Season to taste with salt and pepper.

3. To serve, spoon into bowls, top with a generous dollop or two of yogurt, and sprinkle with parsley.

PER ⅙ RECIPE
Calories: 154
Dietary fiber:
5 grams
Protein: 10 grams
Carbohydrates:
24 grams
Good fats: 2 grams
Other fats: <1 gram

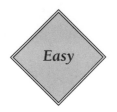

SERVES 6

Pasta and Mushroom Chowder

Bonnie Bruce

This soup combines the complementary textures of pasta and mushrooms. The carrots and yams add important protective nutrients and a creamy richness to the soup. Don't skimp on the exotic mushrooms—they make the soup especially pleasing and tasty.

1 tablespoon extra virgin olive oil
1 medium onion, chopped
2 cups quartered fresh button mushrooms
1 medium carrot, scrubbed or peeled and diced
1 small red garnet yam, peeled and diced
2 tablespoons whole wheat flour
8 cups Simple Vegetable Stock (page 207)
6 to 8 dried porcini mushrooms (or stemmed, dried shiitake
    mushrooms), rinsed
1 cup tricolor pasta twists, uncooked
Salt and freshly ground pepper
Plain nonfat or lowfat yogurt without gelatin or thickeners
    (optional)

PER SERVING
Calories: 174
Dietary fiber:
3 grams
Protein: 7 grams
Carbohydrates:
32 grams
Good fats: 2 grams
Other fats: <1 gram

1. In a large soup pot, gently warm the oil. Add onion, button mushrooms, diced carrot and yam pieces. Cook over moderate heat, stirring frequently, until vegetables are tender, about 10 minutes.

2. Sprinkle flour over vegetables. Stir to coat and cook for 1 more minute, stirring constantly. Add 1 cup of stock and stir to blend.

3. Add remaining stock to pan. Stir in rinsed, dried mushrooms and uncooked pasta. Bring to a boil. Cook for 8 to 10 more minutes or until pasta is cooked. Season to taste with salt and pepper. Serve topped with plain yogurt if desired.

Red Lentil Soup with Fresh Greens

Bonnie Bruce

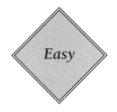

Easy

SERVES 4 TO 6

Red lentils are an appetizing and appealing choice because they give a beautiful color to soups and stews and are among the most easily digested of the legumes. The spinach and tomatoes contribute additional healing and protective nutrients and add to this soup's overall flavor and texture.

2 tablespoons extra virgin olive oil
1½ cups chopped onion
3 large cloves garlic, peeled and chopped
1 teaspoon dried thyme leaves
1 teaspoon dried marjoram leaves
2 cups red lentils, uncooked
2 ripe, medium-size tomatoes, chopped
5 cups thinly sliced fresh spinach leaves
Salt and freshly ground pepper

1. In a soup pot, gently warm the olive oil. Cook the onion and garlic over moderate heat until translucent, about 10 minutes.

2. Stir in thyme, marjoram, lentils, and tomatoes. Add 5½ cups water. Bring to a boil, then lower heat and simmer, partially covered, until lentils are tender, about 15 to 20 minutes.

3. When lentils are cooked, stir in the spinach leaves and simmer for a few more minutes until leaves are just wilted but still bright green. Season to taste with salt and pepper.

PER ⅙ RECIPE
Calories: 292
Dietary fiber:
11 grams
Protein: 20 grams
Carbohydrates:
44 grams
Good fats: 4 grams
Other fats: <1 gram

Ziti and Cannellini Hot Pot

Bonnie Bruce

SERVES 3 TO 4

Traditionally known as the Italian soup pasta e fagioli, *this version is made exclusively with fresh foods from plants. If beans seem a little heavy right now, put them through a ricer first to remove the skins. Or, if preferred, omit the beans altogether.*

1 tablespoon extra virgin olive oil
1 cup chopped onion
½ cup chopped fresh tomatoes
3 cups water or Simple Vegetable Stock (page 207)
¼ cup tomato paste
2 cloves garlic, peeled and minced
¼ teaspoon crushed red pepper (optional)
¼ cup chopped fresh Italian parsley
1 bay leaf
1 teaspoon chopped dried rosemary leaves
¾ cup ziti (or other tube shaped pasta) made from whole
    wheat or 100% durum wheat semolina flour, uncooked
2 cups cooked cannellini or small white beans
Salt and freshly ground pepper

1. Gently warm oil in a large soup pot. Cook onion over moderate heat until tender, about 5 minutes.

2. Add tomatoes, water or stock, tomato paste, garlic, crushed red pepper, parsley, bay leaf, and rosemary. Stir to combine and bring to a boil. Then add the pasta and cook over medium heat until pasta is al dente, about 7 to 10 minutes, stirring occasionally. Check soup during cooking, and add more water or stock if it gets too thick.

PER ¼ RECIPE:
Calories: 268
Dietary fiber:
9 grams
Protein: 12 grams
Carbohydrates:
46 grams
Good fats: 3 grams
Other fats: 1 gram

3. Add beans (or beans that have been riced) and heat through. Remove bay leaf before serving. Season to taste with salt and pepper. Serve piping hot with warm whole grain rolls.

VARIATION

Use diced firm tofu in place of the beans for an easy-to-eat and digest, high quality protein main dish.

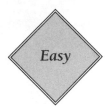

Barley and Friends

Bonnie Bruce

SERVES 4 TO 5

This soup has a slightly chewy texture that comes in part from the easily digestible grain, barley. The friendliness comes from the golden color of red lentils, which also adds to its texture, as well as the mushrooms, which give a bit of variety to this delightful and mild flavored soup. In addition, this is a good soup to make ahead since it freezes well and reheats nicely in the microwave.

1 tablespoon extra virgin olive oil
1 medium onion, coarsely chopped
1 bay leaf
4 cups (½ pound) quartered mushrooms
½ cup red lentils, uncooked
½ cup hulled or whole barley, uncooked
1 ripe, medium-size tomato, diced
4 to 5 cups water or Simple Vegetable Stock (page 207)
3 tablespoons tamari sauce
Salt and freshly ground pepper

1. Gently warm oil in a soup kettle. Cook onion, bay leaf, and mushrooms over moderate heat until onion is translucent, about 5 minutes.

2. Stir in lentils, barley, and tomato. Add water or stock and tamari sauce.

3. Bring to a boil. Stir. Then simmer covered for 45 to 60 minutes, until lentils are creamy and barley is cooked. Check soup during cooking time and add more water or stock if it gets too thick. Remove bay leaf before serving. Season to taste with salt and pepper.

PER ¼ RECIPE
Calories: 251
Dietary fiber:
9 grams
Protein: 15 grams
Carbohydrates:
41 grams
Good fats: 3 grams
Other fats: <1 gram

Mediterranean Minestrone Pronto

Bonnie Bruce

Hearty

SERVES 6

This is a simplified, plant-based version of a classic recipe for minestrone. We've strived to make its preparation as uncomplicated as possible without compromising all the rich sources of healing and protective nutrients that go into it. The recipe makes a big batch, but it freezes well for quick reheating. If beans are hard to digest right now, put them through a ricer first to remove the skins, or, if preferred, omit them altogether.

2 tablespoons extra virgin olive oil
1½ cups chopped leeks, white part only
1 clove garlic, peeled and chopped
6 cups water or Simple Vegetable Stock (page 207)
½ cup tomato paste
1 *each* potato, carrot, and tomato, all diced (peeled, if desired)
1 cup fresh wide green beans, cut into 1-inch pieces
½ teaspoon *each* dried sage and dried oregano leaves
2 cups thinly sliced fresh spinach leaves
1 to 2 cups cooked cannellini or small white beans (optional)
½ cup uncooked pasta tubes, such as penne (whole wheat or
    100% durum wheat semolina flour)
Salt and freshly ground pepper

1. Gently warm the oil in a large soup pot. Cook the leeks and garlic over moderate heat, stirring occasionally until tender, about 10 minutes.

2. Add water or vegetable stock, tomato paste, diced potato, carrot, tomato, green beans, sage, and oregano. Stir to combine. Bring to a gentle boil. Cover and cook over low heat for 20 to 30 minutes, until vegetables are tender but not overcooked.

3. Bring soup to a boil. Stir in spinach, beans, and pasta. Continue simmering for 7 to 10 minutes or until pasta is *al dente*. Add salt and pepper to taste.

PER SERVING
Calories: 232
Dietary fiber:
8 grams
Protein: 11 grams
Carbohydrates:
38 grams
Good fats: 4 grams
Other fats: <1 gram

Hearty

MAKES
10 CUPS

Hearty Green Lentil Soup Provençal

Rowena Hubbard

The small green French du Pay lentils hold their shape and their texture in this hearty microwaveable soup. Combined with red bell peppers, garbanzo beans, tomatoes, and herbs, the flavors are reminiscent of the sunny South of France. Herbs de Provençe is an aromatic blending of thyme, lavender, basil, savory, marjoram, and tarragon. If you can't find the mixture use regular thyme or a mixture of regular thyme and lemon thyme as a substitute.

1 tablespoon extra virgin olive oil
1 cup finely chopped onion
2 cloves garlic, peeled and minced
1 cup small green French du Pay lentils, uncooked
1½ cups cooked cannellini or small white beans
1 cup chopped celery
1 cup diced red bell pepper
4 large very ripe tomatoes, diced
1 teaspoon Herbs de Provençe
Salt and freshly ground pepper

1. Gently warm oil in a soup kettle. Cook onion and garlic over moderate heat until onion is soft. Stir in lentils and beans, and cook until they are well coated with oil.

2. Add celery, diced red pepper, tomato pieces, 4 cups of water, and Herbs de Provençe. Bring to a boil, cover, and turn heat down to simmer. Cook 30 to 45 minutes until lentils are tender but still firm. Season to taste with salt and pepper.

PER 1-CUP
SERVING
Calories: 138
Dietary fiber:
5 grams
Protein: 8 grams
Carbohydrates:
22 grams
Good fats: 2 grams
Other fats: <1 gram

MICROWAVE METHOD

In a large glass bowl, stir together oil, onion, and garlic. Micro-wave, uncovered, on high for 4 minutes. Stir in remaining ingre-dients with 4 cups of water. Cover tightly with plastic wrap and cook on high for 25 minutes. Allow to stand covered for 5 min-utes before serving.

VARIATION

For a soup that's easier to eat and digest, use red lentils and omit the beans and red bell pepper. Also, try different kinds of beans, such as garbanzo beans.

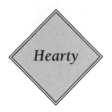

Miso Soup with
Buckwheat Noodles and Beans

Rowena Hubbard

SERVES 4

This miso soup is hearty and very colorful. Use any miso here, dark red if you like a rich strong flavor, light colored if you prefer a mild flavor. Use a very large glass bowl to prepare this soup in the microwave. The noodles tend to make the mixture boil up with large frothy bubbles, so you need lots of space in the cooking bowl. If you cut the recipe in half, the cooking time will be reduced to about 8 minutes.

> 4 ounces dried buckwheat "soba" noodles, broken in half
> 1 cup shredded carrots, peeled if desired
> ½ cup cooked cannellini or small white beans
> 1 tablespoon soy sauce
> 4 to 6 ounces soft tofu (about ⅔ cup), chopped or cut into small cubes
> 3 tablespoons miso
> 2 tablespoons finely minced scallions (green onions)

1. Combine 3 cups water, the broken buckwheat noodles, carrots, beans, and soy sauce in a large (about 6 quarts) glass bowl.

2. Cover tightly with microwaveable plastic wrap. Microwave on high for 12 minutes, turning bowl once halfway through cooking. When mixture is cooked, gently stir in tofu.

3. Blend miso with 3 tablespoons water and swirl into the soup with the scallions. Adjust seasoning, adding another tablespoon of soy sauce if desired, before serving.

PER SERVING
Calories: 130
Dietary fiber:
4 grams
Protein: 8 grams
Carbohydrates:
20 grams
Good fats: 2 grams
Other fats: <1 gram

Chapter 11

PERFECTLY PASTA
AND GREAT GRAINS

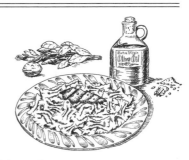

TRADITIONALLY APPEALING AND FOR MANY A COMFORT food, pasta is a reliable and good source of energy, protein, and healthful nutrients. Pastas made from whole wheat flour are among the superstars in the pasta world. They contain all of nature's goodness naturally wrapped up in the unprocessed whole grain kernel, most of which is removed when whole wheat is made into white flour.

Pastas made with soy flour and with wheat germ added are also high in protein. Green and red pastas like those made from spinach and beets add variety, which may be important for sparking your appetite, but add little in the way of vital nutrients. When you do use whole wheat pasta expect a toothsome texture and a full flavor that isn't typical of white flour pasta.

If your digestive tract is sensitive right now, and whole wheat pasta is not suitable or appealing, choose pasta made from 100 percent durum wheat semolina flour. It's higher in protein than plain refined white flour, but remember that it is still a refined product which has had many of its healthful components removed during processing.

In this section, you'll also find recipes for other wholesome grains, like brown rice, wild rice, whole wheat couscous, and millet. Many are filling, make substantial main dishes, and all will add important healing and protective compounds to your diet. Here, too, if your digestive tract is sensitive, we have included variations so that you can use a refined grain (like white rice) until you're feeling better.

Pointers for preparing pastas and grains:

• For best results, cook pasta in a large amount of water that is at a rolling boil before adding pasta. Don't rinse pasta after cooking if you are going to have it with a warm sauce. Do rinse it when you're going to serve it as cold salad to cool it off and stop the cooking.

• Pasta can be cooked to different stages of tenderness. The preferred method is to cook it until it's *al dente,* that is, until it's still a bit chewy—although it can be cooked until softer so that it's easier to eat. Cooking time will depend on how much water you use, the altitude (takes longer at higher altitudes), the pasta shape (angel hair pasta can cook in a minute or two, while rigatoni takes upward of 9 to 10 minutes), and how tender you want it.

• Note that whole grains will take longer to cook, typically sometimes twice as long as their refined counterparts. Directions are given with each recipe. Remember to plan ahead for a longer cooking time.

Supereasy recipes are smooth sippable foods for ease in swallowing without need to chew.

Easy recipes are soft and tender, need some chewing but are gentle on the digestive tract.

Hearty recipes are most suitable when you are feeling well and back to normal.

Recipe	Supereasy	Easy	Hearty
Whole Wheat Couscous with Mushrooms (*page 136*)		◆	
Millet and Carrot Pilaf (*page 138*)		◆	
Linguine with Asparagus, Portabello Mushrooms and Ginger (*page 139*)		◆	
Yogurt Pesto on a Bed of Butterflies (*page 140*)		◆	
Easy Lasagna with Fresh Greens (*page 142*)		◆	
Rigatoni, Tomatoes, and Tofu with an Italian Flair (*page 144*)		◆	
Twisted Noodle Salad (*page 146*)		◆	
Capellini with Fresh Basil, Avocado and Tomatoes (*page 148*)		◆	
Spaghettini with Baked Garlic and Fresh Shitake Mushrooms (*page 149*)		◆	
Brown Rice Pilaf with Apples and Sun-Dried Raisins (*page 150*)		◆	
Fettucine with Creamy Red Lentils and Tomatoes (*page 151*)		◆	
Lentils and Noodles in a Cheesy-Yogurt Sauce (*page 152*)		◆	◆
Medley of Rices with Pumpkin Seeds (*page 154*)		◆	◆
Ragout of Brown Rice, Yams, Tomatoes, and Beans (*page 155*)		◆	◆

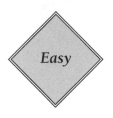

Easy

Whole Wheat Couscous with Mushrooms

Bonnie Bruce

SERVES 4 TO 6

Couscous, made from semolina wheat, is a traditional food of North Africa. Be sure to buy the whole wheat variety to get all the nutrients that are in the whole grain. Couscous is very mild flavored, so this recipe is tastiest when made with the vegetable stock. Try varying the recipe using different kinds of seasonings and different types of mushrooms.

1 tablespoon extra virgin olive oil
3 green onions, including green part, sliced thin
1 cup thinly sliced mushrooms (try fresh shiitakes, brown criminis, or common button mushrooms)
1 to 2 teaspoons dried basil or thyme
2 cups water or Simple Vegetable Stock (page 207)
1 cup uncooked whole wheat couscous
Salt and freshly ground pepper

1. Gently warm the oil in a 2-quart pan with a lid. Cook green onions over low heat for about 5 minutes. Add mushrooms and basil or thyme. Continue to cook over low heat until mushrooms are tender, stirring frequently, about 10 minutes.

2. Add water or vegetable stock and bring to a boil. Add couscous, stir, and return to a boil. Turn off heat, cover, and let sit for 5 minutes. Fluff with a fork. Season to taste with salt and pepper.

PER ½ RECIPE
Calories: 235
Dietary fiber:
3 grams
Protein: 8 grams
Carbohydrates: 44
grams
Good fats: 3 grams
Other fats: <1 gram

VARIATIONS

• Boost the nutritional value by adding cooked cubes of sweet potato or cooked carrot coins to the cooked mushrooms.

• Make a sweeter version by using ½ yellow onion in place of green onions, ⅛ teaspoon powdered saffron, and ½ teaspoon *each* ground ginger, cinnamon, and turmeric for seasoning instead of basil or thyme.

• Couscous also makes a fine breakfast food by preparing it plain with water and adding honey and raisins as desired.

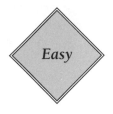

SERVES 4 TO 6

Millet and Carrot Pilaf

Bonnie Bruce

Millet is very mild flavored, easily digested, tender, and rich in both protein and iron. This recipe can be prepared very rapidly. Serve it as a main dish with freshly steamed spinach for a colorful and easy-to-fix meal.

1 tablespoon extra virgin olive oil
½ medium onion, chopped
1 carrot, scrubbed and chopped
1 cup uncooked millet
Salt and freshly ground pepper

1. Gently warm the oil in a medium saucepan. Cook onion and carrot over low to moderate heat until tender, stirring occasionally, about 15 minutes.

2. Add millet and 2 cups of water to the saucepan. Bring to a boil. Stir. Then simmer gently for about 15 minutes, until all water has been absorbed and the millet is tender. Season to taste with salt and pepper.

VARIATIONS

PER ⅕ RECIPE
Calories: 321
Dietary fiber:
4 grams
Protein: 9 grams
Carbohydrates:
60 grams
Good fats: 4 grams
Other fats: 1 gram

• Add ¼ cup sun-dried raisins and/or ½ cup chopped walnuts at the end of cooking.

• Add 1 teaspoon mild curry powder to onion and carrots. Then add ½ cup *each* sun-dried raisins and chopped walnuts at the end of cooking.

Linguine with Asparagus, Portobello Mushrooms, and Ginger

Bonnie Bruce

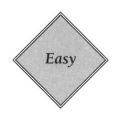

Easy

Typically a welcome sign of spring, tender and green fresh asparagus is complemented by Italian portobello mushrooms with the slight accent of ginger. You can make this pasta dish softer and easier to eat by cooking the vegetables and pasta to desired tenderness. Note that if you use wine, there will be a small amount of alcohol remaining after cooking.

1 tablespoon extra virgin olive oil

1 pound fresh asparagus, trimmed of tough bases and cut into 1½-inch diagonal slices

½ cup green onions, sliced thin diagonally

1 cup portobello mushrooms, quartered and cut into ¼-inch slices

1 clove garlic, peeled and chopped

2 teaspoons peeled and minced fresh ginger

¼ teaspoon crushed red pepper (optional)

¼ cup water or white wine

Salt and freshly ground pepper

4 ounces cooked linguine (whole wheat or 100% durum wheat semolina flour), drained and kept warm

1. Gently warm the oil. Cook the asparagus, green onions, mushrooms, and garlic over moderate heat until crisp tender, about 10 minutes.

2. Stir in ginger, crushed red pepper (if using), and water or wine. Simmer until vegetables are cooked to desired tenderness. Salt and pepper to taste.

3. Toss with pasta and serve immediately.

PER SERVING*
Calories: 418 (448)
Dietary fiber:
16 grams (9 grams)
Protein: 21 grams
(19 grams)
Carbohydrates:
88 grams
(90 grams)
Good fats: 1 gram
(1 gram)
Other fats: <1 gram
(<1 gram)

Made with whole wheat pasta (semolina pasta in parentheses).

Yogurt Pesto on a Bed of Butterflies

Bonnie Bruce

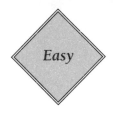

Easy

SERVES 4

In contrast to traditional pesto sauce, this one takes on a more healthful profile by being high in protein. It is a somewhat lighter kind of pesto, but one that is just as flavorful and appealing. It comes out smoother in texture and a creamier green color when made in a blender rather than a food processor.

2 cups firmly packed fresh basil leaves
3 to 4 medium cloves garlic, peeled and left whole
2 tablespoons pine nuts or walnuts
2 tablespoons extra virgin olive oil
½ cup plain nonfat or lowfat yogurt without gelatin or
    thickeners
Nonfat or 1% lowfat milk for thinning pesto
Salt
8 ounces cooked bow-tie (farfalle) pasta (whole wheat or
    100% durum wheat semolina flour), drained and kept warm

PER SERVING*
Calories: 364 (368)
Dietary fiber:
8 grams (3 grams)
Protein: 14 grams
(13 grams)
Carbohydrates:
59 grams
(61 grams)
Good fats: 7 grams
(7 grams)
Other fats: 1 gram
(1 gram)

———

*Made with whole wheat pasta (semolina pasta in parentheses).

1. Put basil, garlic, nuts, and olive oil into a food processor or blender. Blend until a thick paste is formed, about 2 to 3 minutes, scraping sides down as needed.

2. Add yogurt and continue blending until evenly green in color. Add a small amount of milk if you would like a thinner sauce. Season to taste with salt. Spoon attractively over the cooked pasta. Serve immediately.

Note: Leftover pesto sauce can be stored covered in the refrigerator for about a week. The top layer may discolor due to exposure to the air. To take care of this, stir before using.

VARIATIONS

• For added vitamin E and other valuable nutrients, top the pasta and pesto with chopped walnuts before serving.

• Try the pesto on top of a baked potato for a light meal or snack.

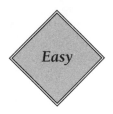

Easy

SERVES 6 TO 8

Easy Lasagna with Fresh Greens

Bonnie Bruce

This recipe is made easy, because you don't have to precook the lasagna noodles. To make the recipe work, though, be sure to use exactly 9 noodles and the exact amount of liquid. To simplify the recipe preparation further, you can substitute 4 cups of the Simply Perfect Tomato Sauce (page 208) for the sauce recipe here. We've also included some tender cooked greens to boost the content of healing and protective nutrients. If you choose to add the richness of the red wine, note that there will be a small amount of alcohol remaining after cooking.

PER ⅙ RECIPE*
Calories: 249 (253)
Dietary fiber:
5 grams (3 grams)
Protein: 16 grams
(15 grams)
Carbohydrates:
35 grams
(37 grams)
Good fats: 2 grams
(2 grams)
Other fats: 3 grams
(3 grams)

*Made with whole wheat pasta (semolina pasta in parentheses).

4 cups diced ripe, medium-size tomatoes
2 cloves garlic, peeled and left whole
1 teaspoon dried basil leaves
¼ cup tomato paste
½ cup water or red wine
Salt and freshly ground pepper
1½ cups part skim ricotta cheese
½ cup nonfat or lowfat yogurt without gelatin or thickeners
1 large whole egg or 2 egg whites
1 teaspoon dried oregano leaves
9 uncooked lasagna noodles (whole wheat or 100% durum wheat semolina flour)
4 cups fresh spinach leaves, steamed or microwaved until wilted, with juices

1. Preheat oven to 350 degrees. Put the tomatoes, garlic, basil, and tomato paste in a blender or food processor and blend until smooth, scraping down sides as needed. Pour into a saucepan, add water or wine, then bring to a boil. Reduce heat and simmer

over moderate heat for 30 minutes. Season sauce to taste with salt and pepper. You will need to have 4 cups of sauce when done. Add water, if needed.

2. Combine the ricotta cheese, yogurt, egg, and oregano in a small bowl. Lightly oil an 8 × 12-inch baking dish. Then ladle ½ cup of sauce over bottom of baking dish. Tilt to cover the bottom with sauce. Top with 3 uncooked lasagna noodles. Spread half of the cheese mixture over the noodles. Then place half of the wilted spinach leaves (undrained) over the cheese mixture. Ladle another ½ cup of the sauce over this layer. Repeat with a second layer. Then top with last 3 noodles and ladle rest of sauce over them.

3. Pull middle oven rack about halfway out of oven being careful not to burn yourself. Put lasagna pan on rack and leave rack pulled out. Pour one cup of water around the edges of the lasagna. Cover pan tightly with foil and slowly push rack into oven. Bake for 40 to 45 minutes or until noodles are tender.

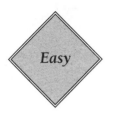
Easy

Rigatoni, Tomatoes, and Tofu with an Italian Flair

Bonnie Bruce

SERVES 6

A mixture of high quality protein and nutrient-rich vegetables combine to make a satisfying and flavorful main dish in this recipe. In addition, the sauce also purees into a smooth and creamy texture, making it easier to eat. Note that if you use the red wine, there will be a small amount of alcohol remaining after cooking.

2 tablespoons extra virgin olive oil

1 medium onion, finely chopped

2 cups thinly sliced mushrooms

1 stalk celery, thinly sliced

1 medium carrot, scrubbed or peeled and chopped

1 package (14 to 16 ounces) firm tofu, cut into ½-inch cubes or crumbled

10 to 12 ripe, medium-size tomatoes, chopped (1 28-ounce can of good quality diced tomatoes *with* liquid may be substituted)

½ cup water or red wine

1 can (6 ounces) tomato paste

3 tablespoons soy sauce

1 bay leaf

1 teaspoon *each* dried basil and oregano leaves

8 ounces cooked rigatoni pasta (whole wheat or 100% durum wheat semolina flour), drained and kept warm

Chopped fresh parsley for garnish

PER SERVING*
Calories: 372 (376)
Dietary fiber:
10 grams (7 grams)
Protein: 17 grams
(16 grams)
Carbohydrates:
58 grams
(60 grams)
Good fats: 7 grams
(7 grams)
Other fats: 1 gram
(1 gram)

———

*Made with whole wheat pasta (semolina pasta in parentheses).

1. Gently heat oil in a large sauce pan. Cook onion, mushrooms, celery, carrot, and tofu together over moderate heat until tender, about 10 to 15 minutes.

2. Stir in tomatoes, water or red wine, tomato paste, soy sauce, bay leaf, basil, and oregano. Bring to a boil. Then simmer over low heat for about 30 minutes or until desired thickness, stirring frequently. Remove bay leaf before serving. Pour sauce over cooked pasta. Garnish with chopped fresh parsley. Serve immediately.

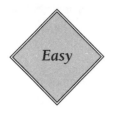

Easy

SERVES 4

Twisted Noodle Salad

Bonnie Bruce

Any time of the year, pasta and fresh vegetables make an appetizing main dish salad. Served cold during the warm months, pasta salad is a refreshing change from a traditional hot entree. To make this recipe easier to eat, vegetables such as carrots and summer squash could be cooked first to soften them. The less easily digestible ingredients like cucumber and olives could also be omitted.

Salad ingredients

    1 medium raw carrot, scrubbed or peeled and chopped

    1 small cucumber, peeled and diced

    1 small crookneck squash, chopped

    ¼ cup (5 to 6 large) pitted, chopped, oil-cured or dried olives (like Greek or Italian)

    ¼ cup chopped fresh Italian parsley, plus additional parsley for garnish

    2 ripe, medium-size tomatoes, diced

    3½ cups cooked tri-color rotini pasta (whole wheat or 100% durum wheat semolina flour), rinsed in cold water and drained

Dressing ingredients

    3 tablespoons extra virgin olive oil

    1 tablespoon balsamic vinegar

    1 garlic clove, peeled and minced

    ½ teaspoon dried basil leaves

    Salt and freshly ground pepper

PER SERVING*
Calories: 400 (408)
Dietary fiber:
10 grams (5 grams)
Protein: 12 grams
(11 grams)
Carbohydrates:
61 grams
(64 grams)
Good fats: 10 grams
(10 grams)
Other fats: 2 grams
(2 grams)

*Made with whole wheat pasta (semolina pasta in parentheses).

1. Combine all the salad ingredients together.

2. In a jar with a lid, shake together the olive oil, vinegar, garlic, and basil leaves to make dressing. Season to taste with salt and pepper.

3. Pour dressing over pasta and vegetables and gently toss to combine. Garnish with additional parsley. Serve at room temperature or chilled.

VARIATIONS

• Vary flavors by using different kinds of fresh vegetables in season, like summer squash, radishes, celery, or small broccoli florets.

• Add a diced ripe avocado for added richness and flavor.

• For added zest, add 1 tablespoon drained capers with the salad ingredients.

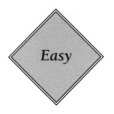

Easy

Capellini with Fresh Basil, Avocados, and Tomatoes

Bonnie Bruce

SERVES 4

Particularly during the summer when vine ripened tomatoes and fresh basil are readily available, this is a perfect entree for a light meal. To make this easier to eat, the tomatoes could be pureed first.

2 tablespoons extra virgin olive oil

2 cloves garlic, peeled and minced

1 cup fresh basil leaves, chopped

½ to ¾ large Haas avocado, peeled and cut into small cubes

4 ripe, medium-size tomatoes, cut into small cubes

12 ounces cooked capellini or angel hair pasta (whole wheat or 100% durum wheat semolina flour), drained and kept warm

Salt and freshly ground pepper

PER SERVING*
Calories: 420 (428)
Dietary fiber:
13 grams (6 grams)
Protein: 13 grams
(12 grams)
Carbohydrates:
65 grams
(68 grams)
Good fats: 10 grams
(10 grams)
Other fats: 2 grams
(2 grams)

———

*Made with whole wheat pasta (semolina pasta in parentheses).

1. Gently warm oil in a pan large enough to mix the cooked pasta with the avocado and tomatoes. Add garlic to the oil and simmer for about 5 minutes, not allowing the garlic to brown.

2. Remove the pan from heat. Add chopped basil, avocado, and tomatoes to the pan. Add cooked pasta and gently toss to combine. Season to taste with salt and pepper. Serve immediately.

VARIATION

For added zest, before adding vegetables to pan, pour 1 to 2 tablespoons of balsamic vinegar into the bottom of the pan and toss with the pasta.

Spaghettini with Baked Garlic and Fresh Shiitake Mushrooms

Bonnie Bruce

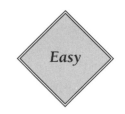

Easy

SERVES 4

Spaghettini noodles are thinner than regular spaghetti, and they complement the texture of shiitake mushrooms well. The baked garlic adds a mild flavor and a creaminess to the dish. The carrots and tomatoes are rich sources of carotenoids and other phytochemicals, and with the garlic, are important for healing.

2 tablespoons extra virgin olive oil

2 medium carrots, scrubbed or peeled and cut into
   2-inch matchsticks

3 to 4 medium-sized fresh shiitake mushrooms, sliced
   ½-inch thick

1 medium zucchini, cut into 2-inch matchsticks

2 heads baked garlic (page 211)

2 teaspoons dried basil leaves

Salt and freshly ground pepper

8 ounces cooked spaghettini (whole wheat or 100% durum
   wheat semolina flour), drained and kept warm

1 fresh, medium-size tomato, diced

1. Warm the oil in a medium pan and cook carrots, mushrooms, and zucchini for 2 to 3 minutes or until just barely tender. Don't overcook; they should have a slight crunch to them.

2. Squeeze the baked garlic heads into a small bowel. Stir in ⅓ cup water and basil. Add to the vegetables in the pan. Bring to a boil and simmer for a few minutes. Season to taste with salt and pepper. Pour over hot pasta, add the tomato, and toss.

PER SERVING*
*Calories: 375 (387)
Dietary fiber:
10 grams (5 grams)
Protein: 13 grams
(11 grams)
Carbohydrates:
65 grams
(69 grams)
Good fats: 6 grams
(6 grams)
Other fats: 1 gram
(1 gram)*

———

*Made with whole wheat pasta (semolina pasta in parentheses).

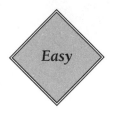

Brown Rice Pilaf with Apples and Sun-Dried Raisins

Bonnie Bruce

SERVES 4

Short grain brown rice gives a creamy texture to this wholesome combination of rice and fruit, while the apples and raisins boost the health-enhancing phytochemicals (see page 11). Vary the sweetness and flavor by substituting different apple varieties. For example, use a sweeter tasting Gala apple instead of a tart Granny Smith. If you'd prefer something easier to chew and digest, short grain white rice may be used instead of the brown rice, but reduce cooking time to 15 to 20 minutes.

1 tablespoon extra virgin olive oil
½ cup finely chopped onion
1 cup short grain brown rice, uncooked
1 medium-size Granny Smith apple, peeled, cored, and chopped
¼ cup sun-dried raisins
Salt and freshly ground pepper

PER SERVING*
Calories: 235 (279)
Dietary fiber: 7 grams (5 grams)
Protein: 4 grams (5 grams)
Carbohydrates: 48 grams (58 grams)
Good fats: 3 grams (3 grams)
Other fats: <1 gram (<1 gram)

*Made with brown rice (white rice in parentheses).

1. Gently warm the oil in a medium saucepan with a lid. Cook onion over moderate heat until tender.

2. Add 2 cups water and bring to a boil. Stir in rice and return to a boil. Stir. Then cover and simmer for 30 to 35 minutes.

3. Stir in chopped apple and raisins and simmer covered for another 5 minutes. Season to taste with salt and pepper. Best served warm. Reheats very nicely in a microwave.

VARIATIONS

• Use chopped dates instead of raisins.
• Stir in ½ cup slivered almonds at the end of cooking for added crunch.

Fettucine with Creamy
Red Lentils and Tomatoes

Bonnie Bruce

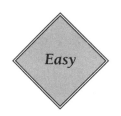

Easy

This is a satisfying entree that is quick to prepare. The red lentils
cook fast and disintegrate during cooking, which gives a creamy texture to the sauce. Feel free to blend or process the sauce after cooking
if you'd prefer it smoother. Remember that if you use the wine, there
will be a small amount of alcohol remaining after cooking.

SERVES 4

1 tablespoon extra virgin olive oil

1 shallot, minced (or ½ medium onion, minced)

½ teaspoon *each* dried oregano leaves and dried basil leaves

1 cup red lentils, uncooked

2 cups ripe tomatoes, cut into small cubes or 2 cups good
   quality, canned diced tomatoes, drained

¼ cup red wine (optional)

Salt and freshly ground pepper

8 ounces cooked fettucine (whole wheat or 100% durum
   wheat semolina flour), drained and kept warm

1. Gently warm the oil in a medium skillet. Cook shallot until
soft over moderate heat, about 5 to 10 minutes.

2. Stir in oregano and basil leaves, red lentils, tomatoes, 2 cups
water, and red wine (if using). Bring to a boil. Reduce heat and
simmer until lentils are very soft, about 20 to 25 minutes. The
longer you simmer the sauce, the smoother and creamier it
becomes. Season to taste with salt and pepper.

3. Pour sauce over cooked pasta and serve immediately.

PER SERVING*
Calories: 501 (509)
*Dietary fiber: 15
grams (10 grams)*
*Protein: 26 grams
(24 grams)*
*Carbohydrates:
88 grams
(92 grams)*
*Good fats: 4 grams
(4 grams)*
*Other fats: 1 gram
(1 gram)*
___
**Made with whole
wheat pasta
(semolina pasta in
parentheses).*

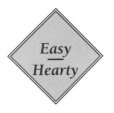

Easy
Hearty

Lentils and Noodles in a Cheesy-Yogurt Sauce

Bonnie Bruce

SERVES 4

The high quality protein in lentils, ricotta cheese, and yogurt make this a hearty main dish casserole. See the variation at the end of the recipe if you'd like an easier-to-digest version without the lentils. The protein content without lentils, though, will be less.

½ cup uncooked brown lentils
½ cup chopped onion
1 medium carrot, scrubbed or peeled and shredded
2 cloves garlic, peeled and chopped
1 tablespoon soy sauce
1½ cups uncooked macaroni (whole wheat or 100% durum wheat semolina flour)
Salt and freshly ground pepper
1½ cups part skim ricotta cheese
½ cup plain nonfat or lowfat yogurt without gelatin or thickeners
1 large whole egg, slightly beaten
1 teaspoon dried oregano leaves
¾ cup nonfat or 1% milk
Paprika and wheat germ for topping

PER SERVING*
Calories: 336 (344)
Dietary fiber:
6 grams (4 grams)
Protein: 24 grams
(24 grams)
Carbohydrates:
42 grams
(44 grams)
Good fats: 3 grams
(3 grams)
Other fats: 5 grams
(5 grams)

———

*Made with lentils and whole wheat pasta (semolina pasta in parentheses).

1. Preheat oven to 350 degrees. Put lentils and 4 cups of water into a soup kettle. Bring to a boil. Add onion, carrot, garlic, and soy sauce. Lower heat and boil gently for 25 to 30 minutes, until lentils and vegetables are tender.

2. Stir the macaroni into the lentil mixture and boil for 5 to 10 minutes more or until tender. Add more water if needed (the

lentils should be cooked by this time). Drain off any extra water. Season to taste with salt and pepper.

3. In a bowl, combine the ricotta cheese, yogurt, egg, oregano, and milk. Then spread half of the lentil-macaroni mixture on the bottom of a lightly oiled or nonstick 9-inch baking dish. Pour half of the ricotta mixture over the macaroni. Repeat with the rest of the lentil-macaroni and ricotta mixtures, ending with the ricotta.

4. Sprinkle top with about a tablespoon each of paprika and wheat germ. Bake for 30 to 35 minutes or until set.

VARIATION

To make this recipe without lentils, simply cook onion, carrot, garlic, and soy sauce as directed, omitting the lentils. Then follow the rest of recipe directions.

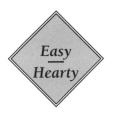

Easy
Hearty

Medley of Rices
with Pumpkin Seeds

Bonnie Bruce

SERVES 6

Brown and wild rices are more healthful choices than white rice, which has had many of its healing and protective substances removed during refining. This high energy, flavorful entree or side dish will be a welcome addition to your diet and is especially suited for when you're feeling well. If you would like to sample its flavors but would prefer a more easily digestible version, long grain white rice can be substituted for both the brown and wild rices—just reduce the cooking time for the white rice to about 20 to 25 minutes.

1 tablespoon extra virgin olive oil
1 medium onion, chopped fine
3 cloves garlic, peeled and chopped
1 cup long grain brown rice, uncooked
½ cup wild rice, uncooked
5¼ cups water or Simple Vegetable Stock (page 207)
¾ cup chopped fresh cilantro
½ cup pumpkin seeds
Salt and freshly ground pepper to taste

PER SERVING*
Calories: 260 (291)
Dietary fiber:
5 grams (3 grams)
Protein: 8 grams
(8 grams)
Carbohydrates:
48 grams
(58 grams)
Good fats: 4 grams
(3 grams)
Other fats: <1 gram
(<1 gram)

*Made with brown rice (white rice in parentheses).

1. Gently warm the oil in a medium saucepan with a lid. Cook onion and garlic over low to moderate heat until tender but without browning, about 10 minutes.

2. Add brown rice and wild rice to pan. Add the water or vegetable stock and bring to a boil, stirring to separate grains. Reduce heat to low. Cover. Cook for 40 to 45 minutes or until rice is cooked and water is absorbed.

3. Remove from heat and let stand for 10 minutes. Stir in cilantro and pumpkin seeds. Season to taste with salt and pepper.

Ragout of Brown Rice, Yams, Tomatoes, and Beans

Bonnie Bruce

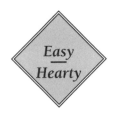

Easy
—
Hearty

SERVES 6

This is a flavorful, hearty, and colorful main dish. Be sure to use short grained rice, which cooks up moist and tender and produces a more stew-like finish. This recipe purees nicely by adding a little water during blending. If you would like to try these flavors in a version that's easier to eat and digest, use short grain white rice, omit the sun-dried tomatoes and beans, and shorten the cooking time to about 20 to 25 minutes.

1 tablespoon extra virgin olive oil

1 medium onion, chopped fine

1 small red garnet yam, cut into ½-inch cubes (about 1 cup)

3 cloves garlic, peeled and chopped

1½ cups short grain brown rice, uncooked

4 cups water or Simple Vegetable Stock (page 207)

1 teaspoon dried oregano leaves

½ teaspoon salt

½ cup (6 to 8 halves) sun-dried tomatoes in olive oil, drained and cut into strips

1 cup cooked garbanzo beans

1. Gently warm the oil in a medium saucepan with a lid. Cook onion, yam pieces, and garlic over moderate heat for about 5 minutes, or until onion is tender (the yam will still be undercooked).

2. Stir in rice, water or vegetable stock, oregano, and salt. Bring to a boil. Then reduce heat, cover, and simmer for 30 minutes. Gently stir in sun-dried tomatoes and beans. Continue to simmer until rice is tender and water is absorbed, about 10 to 20 minutes.

PER SERVING*
Calories: 288 (328)
Dietary fiber: 5 grams (4 grams)
Protein: 9 grams (9 grams)
Carbohydrates: 54 grams (64 grams)
Good fats: 3 grams (3 grams)
Other fats: 1 gram (1 gram)

---

*Made with brown rice (white rice in parentheses).

Chapter 12

VITAL VEGGIE ENTREES

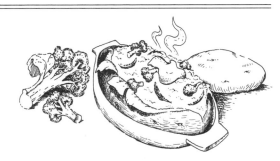

THESE RECIPES FEATURE VEGETABLES THAT WILL NOT ONLY satisfy you, but will also provide the ultimate and optimal sources of restorative and protective phytochemicals. They supply energy (calories)—especially starchy vegetables like potatoes, sweet potatoes, and winter squash—nearly all vitamins and minerals, and some dietary fiber. Some will also contribute significantly to your protein needs when they include cooked dry beans, lentils, or tofu.

Although these recipes accentuate the vegetable as the centerpiece of the meal, don't forget about Stellar Soups and Perfectly Pasta and Great Grain recipes—which call for single vegetables or fuse the flavors of several vegetables with the greatness of grains.

Veggie entrees in this chapter range from the easy-to-eat and easy-to-digest to hearty meals with robust flavors that will tantalize your taste buds. Let these recipes serve as the base for an endless number of variations that you can create, depending on your preferences and seasonal produce availability.

Here are a few tips about veggie main dishes:

• When time and energy allow, garnish your main dishes with chopped parsley, chives, green onions, or tomatoes. Garnishing adds eye-appeal and a finishing touch, which can help spark a dull appetite, as well as add goodness to the recipe itself.

• Veggies offer an endless amount of diversity; there's a wide variety of colors, flavors, and textures. Explore the produce section and be adventurous by trying new ones. The really good news is that when buying vegetables, you can usually just buy one or two pieces to try. You won't have to buy a whole package of something that you're not sure you'll like.

• Note that if your immune system is compromised by treatment, eat only well cooked vegetables that have been thoroughly washed to minimize the risk of infection through the digestive tract. Also, pick thick skinned, peelable varieties until you are stronger.

Vital Veggie Entrees

Supereasy recipes are smooth sippable foods for ease in swallowing without need to chew.

Easy recipes are soft and tender, need some chewing but are gentle on the digestive tract.

Hearty recipes are most suitable when you are feeling well and back to normal.

Recipe	Supereasy	Easy	Hearty
Spaghetti Squash with Tomatoes and Avocado (*page 159*)		◆	
Tofu Stir-Fry with Ginger and Carrots (*page 160*)		◆	
Baked Tubers and Roots with Choice of Legumes (*page 162*)		◆	
Tofu-Mushroom Scramble (*page 164*)		◆	
Mild Curried Spinach and Lentils (*page 165*)			◆
Oven-Baked Veggies with a Yam Canopy (*page 166*)		◆	
Baked Potatoes with Broccoli, Sun-Dried Tomatoes, and Walnuts (*page 168*)			◆

Spaghetti Squash with Tomatoes and Avocado

Bonnie Bruce

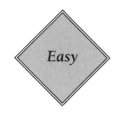

Easy

Also called vegetable spaghetti, this winter squash is rather novel. When cooked, the flesh resembles spaghetti strands; hence its name. It has a mild flavor and a crisp texture which go very well with the creaminess of the avocado and the flavor of the tomato sauce.

1 medium-size Spaghetti Squash
1 recipe Simply Perfect Tomato Sauce (page 208)
1 medium Haas avocado, peeled, seeded, and cut into ½-inch
  cubes
Chives for garnish

1. Preheat oven to 350 degrees. Cut squash in half lengthwise. Remove seeds. Place cut side down on baking sheet and bake for 30 minutes. Turn and continue baking until tender (about 10 to 15 minutes more). Or microwave 10 to 15 minutes in covered dish with ¼ cup water, cut side down.

2. Let squash become cool enough to handle. With fork, remove spaghetti-like strands of squash into serving dish.

3. Heat tomato sauce and gently stir avocado pieces into it. Spoon over squash and serve. Top with freshly chopped chives.

PER SERVING
Calories: 219
Dietary fiber:
6 grams
Protein: 4 grams
Carbohydrates:
26 grams
Good fats: 9 grams
Other fats: 2 grams

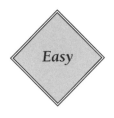

Easy

Tofu Stir-Fry with Ginger and Carrots

Bonnie Bruce

SERVES 4

A mild, temptingly sweet flavored and colorful main dish that goes together quickly, the vegetables in this recipe can be cooked until they are just barely tender or longer, if you prefer them softer. For a version that's easier to digest, omit the red pepper and the almonds. To thicken the sauce we have used arrowroot, a natural fine white powder made from the root of the aru (from the Aruac Indians) rather than the more refined thickener, cornstarch. You should be able to find arrowroot in many supermarkets and health food stores.

1 tablespoon extra virgin olive oil
½ large onion, chopped
2 large carrots, cut into ½-inch-thick diagonal coins
1 red bell pepper, sliced into thin strips
⅔ cup fresh squeezed orange juice
¼ cup honey
2 tablespoons soy sauce
¾ teaspoon chopped fresh ginger
1½ teaspoons arrowroot
1 package (14 to 16 ounces) firm tofu, diced
¼ cup slivered almonds
Hot cooked brown rice

PER SERVING*
Calories: 352
Dietary fiber:
2 grams
Protein: 20 grams
Carbohydrates:
32 grams
Good fats: 14 grams
Other fats: 2 grams
———
*Made with red pepper and almonds.

1. Gently warm the oil in a large skillet. Over moderate heat, stir-fry onion, carrots, and red pepper strips for 5 minutes, or if you'd prefer them very soft, continue to cook to desired tenderness.

2. While vegetables are cooking, whisk together the orange juice, honey, soy sauce, ginger, and arrowroot in a small bowl.

3. Add orange juice mixture and tofu cubes to cooked vegetables and combine gently, making sure tofu and vegetables are coated with the sauce. Cook over medium heat for 1 to 2 minutes until sauce thickens. Stir in almonds just before serving. Serve over hot brown rice.

VARIATION

Add sliced summer squash, mushrooms, or other favorite vegetable combinations with the carrots.

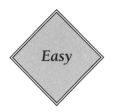

Easy

Baked Tubers and Roots with Choice of Legumes

Bonnie Bruce

SERVES 4 TO 6

This is a beautiful combination of phytochemical-packed, mild-flavored vegetables that are cooked until they are soft and easy to chew. For an easy-to-eat main dish and one that's gentle on your digestive tract, use tofu cubes for your legume choice. For a heartier and more robust version, add the beans toward the end of cooking. You may want to try cannellini and small white beans, which tend to be easier to digest than beans such as kidneys or garbanzos. Or use a variety of different beans for visual and flavor variety.

2 medium carrots, scrubbed and cut into 2-inch pieces
1 medium red garnet yam, peeled if desired, and cut into 2-inch cubes
4 red skinned potatoes, peeled if desired, and cut into 2-inch cubes
2 medium parsnips, peeled and cut into 2-inch pieces
8 large cloves garlic, peeled and left whole
1 package (14 to 16 ounces) firm tofu, cut into 1½-inch cubes or 1½ cups cooked dry beans (e.g., cannellini, small white beans, kidneys, garbanzos, pintos, etc.), kept hot
3 tablespoons extra virgin olive oil
1 tablespoon balsamic vinegar
1 tablespoon dried rosemary leaves
Salt and freshly ground pepper

PER ⅙ RECIPE*
Calories: 267
Dietary fiber:
5 grams
Protein: 8 grams
Carbohydrates:
34 grams
Good fats: 8 grams
Other fats: 1 gram

———

*Made with tofu.

1. Preheat oven to 450 degrees. Combine carrots, yams, red potatoes, parsnips, and garlic cloves in large bowl. Include tofu in this step if using. (Reserve beans for step 4.)

2. Measure oil, vinegar, and rosemary leaves into a small jar with lid. Close tightly and shake to mix. Pour over vegetables and gently toss them to coat evenly.

3. Place vegetables in a single layer, slightly touching is OK, on a nonstick baking pan or one that has been lightly oiled.

4. Bake for 35 to 40 minutes or until vegetables are tender and brown, turning once after 20 minutes. Add beans during the last few minutes of cooking, not allowing them to burn. Remove vegetables to serving platter and serve while hot. Season to taste with salt and pepper.

VARIATIONS

• Vary the vegetables by trying onions, rutabagas, fennel, or celery.

• Vary the seasonings by trying a mild curry powder, a spicy chile powder, or oregano instead of rosemary.

Tofu-Mushroom Scramble

Rowena Hubbard

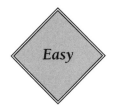

Easy

SERVES 2

Soft tofu makes a wonderfully easy and tasty scramble that's delicious over whole wheat toast for breakfast or over steamed green vegetables (such as asparagus, green beans, kale, Swiss chard, or spinach) as a light lunch or dinner. It is also good over broiled sliced tomatoes. And it's so easy to put together, it can be on the table in under 10 minutes.

1 tablespoon extra virgin olive oil
1 cup sliced fresh mushrooms
½ cup finely minced green onions
1 package (14 to 16 ounces) soft tofu, crumbled
¼ teaspoon turmeric
Salt and freshly ground pepper

1. Gently warm the oil in a large skillet. Cook mushrooms over moderate heat until lightly browned. Stir in green onions and continue to cook until they are wilted.

2. Stir in tofu and sprinkle it with turmeric. Add salt and pepper to taste. Combine gently with mushrooms and green onions, cooking until heated through. Serve immediately.

PER SERVING
Calories: 245
Dietary fiber:
4 grams
Protein: 19 grams
Carbohydrates:
9 grams
Good fats: 14 grams
Other fats: 2 grams

Mild Curried Spinach and Lentils

Rowena Hubbard

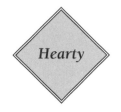

Hearty

SERVES 6

A hearty but mild-flavored and quick casserole that's cooked in the microwave, these lentils keep their shape and have a nice firm bite. If you are used to soft, disintegrating lentils in soups, you'll find these much different. They have an almost crunchy texture. Serve this casserole with steamed vegetables and top it with plain nonfat or lowfat yogurt if you like a little piquant flavor.

1 cup finely chopped onion
2 large cloves garlic, peeled and minced
2 tablespoons extra virgin olive oil
1 teaspoon mild curry powder
1 cup brown lentils, uncooked
½ cup bulgur wheat, uncooked
2 large ripe tomatoes, chopped
1 bunch young spinach leaves (about 4 cups), washed,
   stemmed, and coarsely chopped
Salt and freshly ground pepper

1. Combine onion, garlic, and olive oil in a large glass bowl. Toss lightly to coat with oil. Microwave uncovered on high for 4 minutes. Remove from microwave, stir in curry powder, lentils, and bulgur until coated with oil.

2. Place tomatoes in a 1-quart measure. Add water to fill to the 1-quart marker. Stir into lentil mixture. Cover bowl tightly with plastic wrap and microwave on high for 20 minutes.

3. Remove lentils from microwave, lift plastic, and spread spinach on top of casserole. Recover with plastic wrap and return to microwave for 3 minutes until spinach is wilted.

4. Stir spinach into lentil mixture, recover, and let stand about 2 minutes before serving. Season to taste with salt and pepper.

PER SERVING
Calories: 220
Dietary fiber:
8 grams
Protein: 12 grams
Carbohydrates:
34 grams
Good fats: 4 grams
Other fats: <1 gram

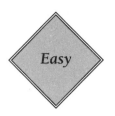

Easy

Oven-Baked Veggies with a Yam Canopy

Bonnie Bruce

SERVES 4

This warming recipe is delicious, chock full of vital nutrients, and satisfying to eat. It also lends itself to the whim of whatever vegetable you may desire or is in season. The yam canopy gives it an engaging, golden-colored, smooth and rich finish. Garnish with bright green, chopped fresh parsley and you'll have a meal fit for a king—a healthy king, that is.

2 tablespoons extra virgin olive oil
1 tablespoon balsamic vinegar
½ teaspoon dried tarragon leaves
1 large onion, peeled and cut into sixths
2 large carrots, scrubbed or peeled and cut into 2-inch pieces
2 medium rutabagas, peeled and cut into 2-inch pieces
2 stalks celery, cut into 2-inch slices (discard leaves)
6 whole cloves garlic, peeled and left whole
1 package (14 to 16 ounces) extra firm tofu, cut into 1-inch cubes
2 pounds red garnet yams, peeled and cut into 2-inch pieces
1 teaspoon powdered ginger
Salt and freshly ground pepper

PER SERVING
Calories: 452
Dietary fiber:
10 grams
Protein: 15 grams
Carbohydrates:
71 grams
Good fats: 10 grams
Other fats: 2 grams

1. Preheat oven to 425 degrees. Shake oil, vinegar, and tarragon together in a small jar. Put onion, carrots, rutabagas, celery, garlic, and tofu into a large bowl. Pour oil and vinegar mixture over them and gently toss to combine. Arrange vegetables in one layer on lightly oiled baking sheet so that they are close together. Bake for 35 minutes, turning after 15 minutes.

2. While vegetables are baking, microwave the yams with 2 tablespoons of water for 10 to 15 minutes, until tender. Mash or whip, using cooking liquid as needed. Stir in ginger. Season to taste with salt and pepper.

3. When vegetables are done to desired tenderness, remove from oven and put them into a baking dish. Spread mashed yams on top. Place under broiler to brown top lightly, about 1 to 2 minutes.

VARIATION

Use dried thyme leaves instead of tarragon for a different flavor.

Hearty

Baked Potatoes with Broccoli, Sun-Dried Tomatoes, and Walnuts

Rowena Hubbard

SERVES 2

This hearty main dish is perfect for those times when you're feeling energetic. It would make a grand lunch or a hearty dinner depending on the size of the potatoes. For a more readily digestible dish, substitute a softer cooked vegetable, like carrots or spinach, or just omit the walnuts. For a finishing touch, top with Yogurt Cheese or plain yogurt.

2 medium to large baking potatoes
1½ cups raw broccoli florets
2 tablespoons chopped sun-dried tomatoes without oil
1 teaspoon dried dill weed
Yogurt Cheese (page 210) or plain nonfat or lowfat yogurt
    without gelatin and thickeners
Salt and freshly ground pepper
2 tablespoons walnuts, toasted and chopped (optional)

1. Preheat oven to 350 degrees. Scrub potatoes well. Pierce several times with a fork and bake for about 50 minutes until soft, or microwave until done.

2. Meanwhile, combine broccoli, sun-dried tomatoes, and dill in a small saucepan. Just before serving add 2 tablespoons water, cover, and steam for 1 to 2 minutes until broccoli is bright green and still crisp.

3. Open baked potatoes and fluff with a fork. Spoon one half of broccoli mixture over each potato. Add salt and pepper to taste. Top with Yogurt Cheese or yogurt and walnuts, if using.

PER SERVING
Calories: 332
Dietary fiber:
8 grams
Protein: 9 grams
Carbohydrates:
65 grams
Good fats: 4 grams
Other fats: <1 gram

Chapter 13

VEGGIES ON THE LIGHT SIDE

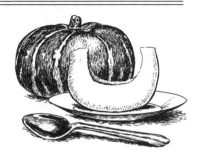

IN OUR CULTURE, THERE IS A "VEGETABLE AS SIDE DISH" mentality—that is, they are pushed to one corner of the plate while other foods take over center stage. However, the "light" dishes in this section make wonderful and satisfying whole meals as well as side dishes. Indeed, if your appetite is waning, these recipes offer you many inviting choices—like the smooth texture of potato puree accented by the mild flavor of baked garlic and the heartier wilted spinach and watercress salad.

Use these recipes as jumping-off points for finding other light and satisfying vegetable combinations that appeal to you. Vegetables can be prepared in an infinite number of ways, from soft or smooth, mild in flavor, and gentle on the digestive tract—to bursting with flavor, texture, heartiness, and robustness.

Whenever there's the opportunity, buy your vegetables from produce stands and farmers' markets where vegetables come directly from the farm. That way they will be as fresh as possible and you'll get the maximum of all of their vitamins, minerals, antioxidants, and protective substances.

Here are a few tips about vegetables on the light side:

• When time or energy is low, simple wilted greens and quick steamed fresh vegetables of any kind are great options. Eat plain, or season as you wish.

• To boost the protein in these vegetable recipes, have a cooked egg, some cottage cheese, or a yogurt smoothie along with it. Or toss in some cubed tofu at the end of cooking. Heartier ways to boost protein include sprinkling nuts and cooked dry beans on top (garbanzos are quite tasty on top of a bed of wilted spinach leaves).

• Remember that when your immune system is compromised by treatment, you should eat only well-cooked vegetables that have been thoroughly washed to minimize the risk of infection through the digestive tract.

Veggies on the Light Side

Supereasy recipes are smooth sippable foods for ease in swallowing without need to chew.

Easy recipes are soft and tender, need some chewing but are gentle on the digestive tract.

Hearty recipes are most suitable when you are feeling well and back to normal.

Recipe	Supereasy	Easy	Hearty
Potato Puree with Baked Garlic (*page 171*)	◆	◆	
Simply Squash (*page 172*)	◆	◆	
Braised Fennel with Carrot Coins (*page 173*)		◆	
Basic Wilted Leafy Greens (*page 174*)		◆	◆
Salad Dressings, Wilted Leafy Green, (*page 176*)		◆	◆
Spinach and Croutons (*page 178*)		◆	
Sweet Chard Stems (*page 179*)		◆	◆
Ginger Savoy (*page 180*)			◆
Collards with Dulse (*page 181*)			◆
Leeks and Kale (*page 182*)			◆
Sweet-Tart Red Kale (*page 183*)			◆
Wilted Spinach and Watercress Salad (*page 184*)			◆

Potato Puree with Baked Garlic

Bonnie Bruce

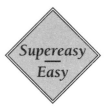

A good source of protein, these potatoes are creamy in texture and easy to eat and digest. If you can find Yukon Gold potatoes, which are creamier and prettier in color than the traditional potatoes used for boiling, they are especially tasty. This recipe can be thinned so that it is sippable, if desired.

1½ pounds boiling potatoes, peeled and cut into 1-inch cubes
1 head Baked Garlic (page 211)
¼ cup nonfat or 1% milk
¼ cup part skim ricotta cheese
Salt and freshly ground pepper
Parsley for garnish

1. Put potatoes into a large saucepan. Cover them with water. Bring to a boil and cook at a low boil for about 20 minutes, or until soft. Drain well.

2. Mash cooked potatoes to desired consistency. They are good either very smooth or with some lumps, if you desire.

3. Squeeze the Baked Garlic onto the potatoes. Stir in the milk and ricotta cheese along with the garlic. Then season to taste with salt and pepper and garnish with fresh chopped parsley.

VARIATIONS

• Top with chopped nuts, such as pistachios.
• Stir in a few tablespoons of chopped sun-dried tomatoes with the cheese and garlic.
• Substitute carrots or red garnet yams for some of the potatoes to give a protective phytochemical boost and a slightly richer flavor.

PER SERVING
Calories: 168
Dietary fiber:
2 grams
Protein: 5 grams
Carbohydrates:
37 grams
Good fats: <1 gram
Other fats: <1 gram

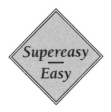

Supereasy — Easy

SERVES 2 TO 4

Simply Squash

Monica Spiller

Two favorite winter squashes are buttercup and kabocha, followed closely by butternut. All of these have a very deep orange colored flesh and are very sweet in flavor. When they are oven baked or microwaved, the sweetness seems to be intensified, and they are so delicious that they can be enjoyed without dressing or accompaniment of any kind. Also, cooked winter squash is very easily mashed or pureed, making it always very easy to eat.

1 winter squash (2 to 3 pounds)

1. Wash and dry the outside of the squash. Pierce it through to the center with a pointed knife in at least four places on the sides. Set it in a microwave-safe dish containing ¼ cup of water. Microwave at full power for approximately 20 minutes, or until the squash is very soft and easily pierced with a fork.

2. Remove squash from oven and cut into quarters. Allow to cool somewhat. Just before serving, remove the seedy center.

3. Serve alone or as a course in between the entree and dessert, to be eaten directly from the skin. Alternatively, scoop the pulp from the skin and serve it, as a vegetable with the main course.

PER ¼ RECIPE
Calories: 132
Dietary fiber:
8 grams
Protein: 3 grams
Carbohydrates:
30 grams
Good fats: <1 gram
Other fats: <1 gram

TO OVEN BAKE A SQUASH

Preheat oven to 425 degrees. Prepare as for the microwave, but bake for one hour or more, until the squash is very soft and can be easily pierced with a fork.

Braised Fennel with Carrot Coins

Bonnie Bruce

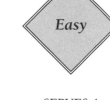

Easy

SERVES 4

The nutrient-rich fennel plant has a delicate sweetness and tenderness that perfectly complements the taste and texture of carrots. This recipe takes little effort to prepare and is delicious hot, warm, or chilled. If you use white wine, note that there will be a small amount of alcohol remaining after cooking.

1 tablespoon extra virgin olive oil
2 bulbs fennel, bottom and tough outer layer removed, then cut into thin slices
2 carrots, scrubbed or peeled and cut into ¼-inch coins
1 teaspoon bouquet garni seasoning (fresh parsley, bay leaf, dried thyme)
¼ cup water or white wine
Salt and freshly ground pepper

1. Gently warm the oil over moderate heat. Cook fennel and carrots over low to moderate heat in a covered pan for about 10 minutes. Turn the vegetables from time to time to prevent browning too much.

2. Stir bouquet garni into vegetables. Add water or wine. Cover and simmer for about 10 to 15 minutes more, until done to desired tenderness. Season to taste with salt and pepper.

VARIATIONS

• Add thinly sliced potatoes with the fennel and carrots.
• Add tomatoes and garlic to vegetables, simmer until tender, and serve over pasta.
• For a different flavoring, replace the bouquet garni with 1 teaspoon *each* dried thyme leaves, marjoram leaves, and tarragon leaves.

PER SERVING
Calories: 79
Dietary fiber:
6 grams
Protein: 2 grams
Carbohydrates:
12 grams
Good fats: 3 grams
Other fats: <1 gram

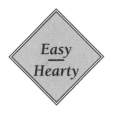

Basic Wilted Leafy Greens

Monica Spiller

The leafy greens are among the prettiest of vegetables and are accepted by all as superfoods full of essential protective nutrients. At the height of their season, they are incredibly sweet and tender. They can then be enjoyed raw when young and sweet, as part of a green salad. And if they are cooked they will often need no dressing at all. Young leaves are usually the most tender. Extra large old leaves tend to be tough.

Leafy greens should be practically free from insect damage. Organic farmers have become very skilled in combating pests in their fields, so if your preference is for organically grown produce, you should be able to have almost blemish and pest free, organically grown leafy greens. If you grow your own leafy greens or are fortunate enough to be able to shop at a local farmer's market, you will have the best chance of having your leafy greens at their peak. Once the greens have been picked, they should be eaten as soon as possible. However, they can be stored in the salad compartment of a refrigerator, for as long as a week provided they are splashed with water.

For variety, and when leafy greens need some help to be appetizing, they can be gently cooked in a little water to the point that they are completely wilted, and then they can be dressed in much the same way as a salad. If you're having digestive problems, spinach and swiss chard are among the easiest of the leafy greens to digest.

1 large bunch leafy greens of choice(about 8 to 12 ounces)

1. *Washing:* Fill a large bowl (8 quarts) with tepid water. Strip and separate the stems from the leafy parts. Tear off damaged leaf areas and discard them. Submerge selected leafy parts in the bowl

of water and allow them to soak for about 5 minutes; this will allow any mud to soften. Swirl the leaves in the water until all the mud has been loosened and has sunk to the bottom of the bowl. Drain the leaves in a colander. Repeat this washing process once or twice more with fresh water, until the water is clean and free from mud. Lift the leaves from the water and allow to drain.

2. *Cooking:* Choose a large saucepan or skillet, 8 to 10 inches in diameter, and add ¼ cup water. Add the washed and drained greens. Set the pan of greens over moderate heat. Bring to a simmer. After a minute or two, as the leaves begin to wilt, gently press them down into the water with a spatula. As soon as the leaves on the bottom have wilted, turn them over so that the top leaves are in the water.

3. When all the leaves have wilted, immediately transfer the greens to a serving dish, so that the bright color is preserved. If the greens are rather tough, drain them and keep the juice. Chop them very finely, and recombine them with the juice in the serving dish.

ACCOMPANIMENTS

• Sweet onions, leeks, and apples are particularly complementary to wilted leafy greens. Leeks with kale is a traditional Scottish combination. Red cabbage with onions, caraway, apple, and vinegar is a popular dish all over northern Europe, but there is no reason why this refreshingly sweet-tart combination cannot also be used with kale instead of red cabbage.

• Use dulse seaweed as a surprising and appetizing accompaniment for leafy greens. Dulse is especially good in the form of small flakes that can be sprinkled onto the wilted greens, or added to a soup with finely chopped kale.

• Spices that transform and complement the flavor of leafy greens, include ginger, black pepper, nutmeg, and caraway. Ginger is used frequently in Chinese cabbage dishes.

PER ½ RECIPE
Calories: 45
Dietary fiber:
6 grams
Protein: 3 grams
Carbohydrates:
10 grams
Good fats: <1 gram
Other fats: <1 gram

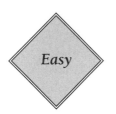

Salad Dressings for Wilted Leafy Greens

Monica Spiller

Choose the ingredients for these salad dressings with care for their quality, flavor, and freshness. Prepare the mixed dressings in a separate bowl. Add them to taste at the table, or toss the greens with the dressing before serving. Season with salt to taste.

Balsamic vinegar, olive oil, and black pepper

Mix 2 to 3 tablespoons olive oil with 1 tablespoon balsamic vinegar and black pepper to taste.

Fresh lemon juice and yogurt

Mix 1 tablespoon freshly squeezed lemon juice with 2 or 3 tablespoons plain nonfat or lowfat yogurt without added gelatin or thickeners.

Honey and balsamic or wine vinegar

Mix 2 tablespoons honey with 2 to 3 tablespoons of the vinegar.

Nutmeg with fresh lemon juice and yogurt

Mix 1 tablespoon freshly squeezed lemon juice with 2 or 3 tablespoons plain nonfat or lowfat yogurt without added gelatin or thickeners. Add ¼ teaspoon freshly grated nutmeg.

Olive oil, red or white wine vinegar, and freshly ground black pepper

Mix 3 tablespoons olive oil with 1 tablespoon wine vinegar. Add pepper to taste.

Olive oil and freshly grated nutmeg

Gently toss cooked greens with a small amount of good quality extra virgin olive oil. Add ¼ teaspoon freshly grated nutmeg.

Olive oil and freshly ground black pepper

Gently toss cooked greens with a small amount of oil and pepper.

Olive oil

Gently toss cooked greens with a small amount of good quality extra virgin olive oil. We suggest about 1 teaspoon of oil per cup of cooked greens.

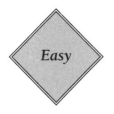

Easy

SERVES 2 TO 4

Spinach and Croutons

Monica Spiller

Spinach is the traditional "super vegetable," well recognized as being very high in protective and healing nutrients. It's also mild in flavor and relatively tender, making it easy on the digestive tract compared to other leafy greens like kale, collards, and cabbage.

> 2 slices whole wheat bread, 1 or 2 days old
> 1 bunch spinach leaves (about 1¼ pounds)
> 1 tablespoon extra virgin olive oil
> Freshly grated nutmeg to taste
> Salt

1. To prepare croutons, preheat oven to 250 degrees. Slice the crust from the bread, and then slice the bread into ½-inch cubes. Spread bread cubes in a single layer, not touching, on a baking stone or tile or a nonstick baking pan. Place them in the oven for 15 to 30 minutes or until they are crispy dry and only slightly browned. Cool on a rack covered with paper.

2. Wash and cook the spinach as described on pages 174–175.

3. Just before serving, toss the spinach with the olive oil and nutmeg. Season to taste with salt. Sprinkle croutons over spinach, and gently toss to combine.

PER ¼ RECIPE
Calories: 92
Dietary fiber:
3 grams
Protein: 4 grams
Carbohydrates:
10 grams
Good fats: 4 grams
Other fats: 1 gram

Sweet Chard Stems

Monica Spiller

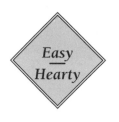

Easy
Hearty

SERVES 2 TO 4

Swiss chard has a distinctive, somewhat mild flavor and a texture similar to spinach, making the two often interchangeable in recipes. You can find chard with either white or red colored stems. In Europe, the stems are often considered to be the prime part of this leafy green. They are distinctively sweet and tender. Serve swiss chard stems along with their wilted greens, as an accompanying side dish, or dress them with one of the dressings suggested on pages 176–177.

Stems from one bunch of red or green swiss chard, ends and damaged parts trimmed, washed, and cut into 1-inch pieces

Add 2 to 3 tablespoons water, to a 6-inch diameter microwaveable dish. Add the chard stems. Cover and microwave for about 3 minutes at high power, or until the stems become soft and translucent.

TO BAKE THE CHARD STEMS

Preheat oven to 375 degrees. Prepare them as for the microwave, then bake for 15 minutes or until they become soft and translucent.

PER ¼ RECIPE
Calories: 36
Dietary fiber:
4 grams
Protein: 4 grams
Carbohydrates:
5 grams
Good fats: <1 gram
Other fats: <1 gram

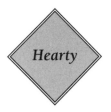

SERVES 2 TO 4

Ginger Savoy

Monica Spiller

The Savoy cabbage is a truly splendid member of the cabbage family, with its deeply crinkled leaves and well rounded form. It has a delicate flavor that contrasts well with the lemony pungency of ginger. Both cabbage and ginger have qualities valuable for cancer prevention and recovery. Serve it as a vegetable side dish or dress the cabbage and ginger as a salad with olive oil, red or white wine vinegar, and a little salt, if desired.

½ head Savoy cabbage, shredded
Peeled and grated fresh ginger root, to taste

1. Put ½ cup water into a medium skillet. Add shredded cabbage and simmer over medium heat until cabbage is translucent and somewhat wilted. Turn the cabbage over with a spatula as the bottom layer becomes wilted.
2. Add ginger to the wilted cabbage. Toss and transfer immediately to a serving dish.

PER ¼ RECIPE
Calories: 36
Dietary fiber:
4 grams
Protein: 2 grams
Carbohydrates:
7 grams
Good fats: <1 gram
Other fats: <1 gram

Collards with Dulse

Monica Spiller

Hearty

SERVES 2 TO 4

On a completely different and perhaps surprising note, dulse is also an appetizing accompaniment for leafy greens. Dulse is an edible sea vegetable (more commonly known as seaweed) that is valuable in its own right as a superfood that provides protein, some soluble fiber, and minerals. Serve this recipe as a vegetable or dress the collards with oil and vinegar and serve as a salad. Since the dulse is salty, additional salt will probably not be needed.

1 bunch collard greens (about 8 to 12 ounces)
1 to 4 tablespoons dulse flakes

1. Wash and cook the collard greens as described for basic greens on page 174.

2. Because collards may be a little tough, after cooking drain them from the saucepan juice, leaving the juice in the pan. Finely chop the greens and then return them to the pan.

3. Sprinkle the dulse flakes over the cooked collards and gently toss to combine. Immediately remove from heat and transfer to a serving dish.

PER ½ RECIPE
Calories: 36
Dietary fiber:
3 grams
Protein: 2 grams
Carbohydrates:
7 grams
Good fats: <1 gram
Other fats: <1 gram

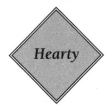

Hearty

SERVES 2 TO 4

Leeks and Kale

Monica Spiller

Kale is available in several different varieties. It can be red, have a gray-green tint, or have different shaped leaves. Whichever you choose, kale provides a wealth of healthful substances, including cancer fighting antioxidants. Serve Leeks and Kale as a vegetable dish or as a salad with any of the dressings suggested on pages 176–177.

1 bunch kale (about 8 to 12 ounces)
1 to 2 leeks

1. Wash and cook the kale as described on pages 174–175. Drain and collect the juice in the same saucepan. Finely chop the kale and set aside.

2. Cut off the tops and bottoms from the leeks, and strip off the tough outermost leaves. Cut the leeks lengthwise down the center, and wash each layer separately. Cut into ½-inch strips.

3. Add the prepared leeks to the saucepan containing the kale juice. Simmer the leeks over moderate heat, for about 3 minutes or until they are just tender and translucent. Add the finely chopped kale. Gently stir together and then remove from heat. Immediately transfer to a serving dish.

PER ½ RECIPE
Calories: 64
Dietary fiber:
3 grams
Protein: 3 grams
Carbohydrates:
13 grams
Good fats: <1 gram
Other fats: <1 gram

Sweet-Tart Red Kale

Monica Spiller

Apples and onions complement the taste and texture of kale and give it a mildly sweet accent. Vary the kind of apple by using a tart Granny Smith, a sweet Gala apple, or one of your favorites. Serve warm as a vegetable or cold as a salad dressed with a little olive oil and red or white wine vinegar.

SERVES 2 TO 4

1 bunch red kale (about 8 to 12 ounces)
1 medium-size cooking apple, peeled, cored, and shredded
1 teaspoon caraway seeds
1 medium sweet yellow onion, peeled and chopped

1. Wash and cook the kale as described on pages 174–175. Drain the kale and collect the juice. Return the juice to the same saucepan. Finely chop the kale and set aside.

2. Add shredded apple and caraway seeds to the saucepan containing the kale juice and simmer for about 3 minutes or until the apples begin to soften.

3. Add the chopped onion to the apples and simmer for another 3 minutes or until the onion is tender and translucent. Stir well and add a little more water if necessary to prevent sticking.

4. Add the chopped kale and gently combine with apple-onion mixture. Remove from heat and transfer to serving dish.

PER ¼ RECIPE
Calories: 76
Dietary fiber:
4 grams
Protein: 3 grams
Carbohydrates:
16 grams
Good fats: <1 gram
Other fats: <1 gram

Hearty

Wilted Spinach and Watercress Salad

Rowena Hubbard

SERVES 2

This knife and fork, salad-side dish, is delicious served hot, cold, or at room temperature. You could use any type of greens and cook them this way (such as bok choy, napa cabbage, beet greens, mustard greens, or Swiss chard). Just be sure that the leaves are young and tender, so that they cook quickly.

1 bunch fresh young spinach (about 8 to 12 ounces)
1 cup young watercress sprigs
1 tablespoon extra virgin olive oil
1 tablespoon fresh squeezed lemon juice
Freshly ground pepper to taste
Cherry tomatoes for garnish

1. Wash spinach and watercress well. Trim roots and long stems from spinach. Place them both in a colander and run water over them, shaking a little, but leaving leaves quite wet.
2. Place greens in a large shallow pan with a tightly fitting lid. Place pan over high heat, and cook until steam begins to escape from under the lid. Check to make sure leaves are wilted. Cooking should take about 3 minutes. Turn into colander to drain; arrange on two salad plates.
3. Drizzle each portion with half the olive oil and then half the lemon juice. Season with freshly ground pepper to taste. Garnish plates with cherry tomatoes to serve.

PER SERVING:
Calories: 90
Dietary fiber:
<1 gram
Protein: 4 grams
Carbohydrates:
5 grams
Good fats: 5 grams
Other fats: 1 gram

Chapter 14

FRUIT AND GRAINS WITH
A SWEET TOUCH

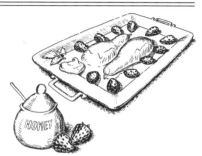

BEFORE THE PERVASIVENESS OF COMMERCIAL BAKED
goods and boxed products, fruit was the conventional way to end
many a meal. In many cultures, fruit still is the traditional way to
end a meal—it cleanses the palate and fulfills that urge to end a
meal with sweetness while giving loads of nutritional dividends.
But best of all, there's no need to limit when you enjoy fruit.
Whenever you're hungry, any time of the day or night, the fruit
recipes in this chapter can be enjoyed.

The wholesome grain recipes in this section are also intended
for you to enjoy at any time. Make a meal out of them when you
just want something simple or a midnight snack. Our versions of
some of the old favorites may be unfamiliar to you, like the rice
pudding with brown rice, but traditionally, before modern food
processing and refining stripped nature's pharmacy nearly bare,
grain dishes were made from the whole grain just as it comes to
us from the soil. We think you'll like the difference and the
wholesome flavors, and we know that you'll benefit from all the
nutritive substances packed in each bit.

A few pointers for enjoying fruits and wholesome grains.

• Buy fruit that is free from blemishes and properly ripe. Produce stands and farmers' markets are often great places to find the best quality and ripest fruits. If you have any question about the ripeness, ask the produce person for assistance. They are usually good resources.

• Grains can be prepared in an almost limitless number of ways. Grains that are gentler on the digestive tract include millet, polenta, whole wheat couscous, and oats. Note that many cooked grains can be thinned to preferred consistency, and can even become sippable as needed.

• Increase protein and calories in cooked grain recipes by adding a quarter cup or more of nonfat dry milk powder to the liquid while cooking.

Fruit and Grains with a Sweet Touch

Supereasy recipes are smooth sippable foods for ease in swallowing without need to chew.

Easy recipes are soft and tender, need some chewing but are gentle on the digestive tract.

Hearty recipes are most suitable when you are feeling well and back to normal.

Recipe	Supereasy	Easy	Hearty
Fifty Ways to Have Hot Grains (*page 188*)	◆	◆	◆
Simply Fruit (Delicious!) (*page 190*)	◆	◆	◆
Fruit Whip with Ricotta Cheese (*page 192*)	◆		
Whole Wheat Couscous with Dates (*page 193*)	◆	◆	
Polenta with Pignolias and Sun-Dried Raisins (*page 194*)	◆	◆	
Quick 'n' Easy Fresh Fruit and Yogurt (*page 195*)		◆	◆
Rice Pudding with Bananas (*page 196*)		◆	
Nectarines and Berries with Yogurt Cheese (*page 197*)		◆	
Sweet Cooked Apple (*page 198*)		◆	
Baked Pears and Peaches with Ginger (*page 199*)		◆	
Vanilla Pears with Strawberries (*page 200*)		◆	
Bread Pudding of the Ancients (*page 202*)		◆	◆
Apple Bake with a Hint of Maple (*page 204*)		◆	

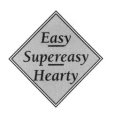

MAKES ABOUT
2 CUPS

Fifty Ways to Have Hot Grains

Bonnie Bruce

Cooked whole grains are naturally rich in healing and protective nutrients. It is proper to have them any time you feel like it—to start up the day, as a snack, or as a light meal. We've given grains a special nutrition boost by adding wheat germ, which contributes a wealth of its own antioxidants, good fats, and other protective substances. You'll also notice that this isn't a traditional recipe. It gives you the basics to design your own appealing combinations.

> 1 cup dry uncooked cereal (mix or match kinds, keeping in mind cooking times)
> $\frac{1}{4}$ cup natural wheat germ
> Salt to taste

Bring $2\frac{1}{4}$ cups water to a boil. Add the grain of your choice. Boil gently for the time given. Stir regularly to keep from sticking to pan.

PER $\frac{1}{2}$-CUP
SERVING*
Calories: 90 to 125
Dietary fiber:
1 to 5 grams
Protein:
1 to 4 grams
Carbohydrates:
15 to 25 grams
Good fats:
<1 to 3 grams
Other fats: <1 gram

*Nutritional value will vary with grain used.

TIPS

• Select whole grains, rather than refined ones to get the maximum nutritional benefit. Look for rolled oats, whole wheat, and stone-ground grains.

• Boost the protein content by adding $\frac{1}{4}$ cup nonfat dry milk powder during cooking.

• If you find temporarily that you need something easier to eat and digest, substitute a refined grain.

• Any of these cereals can be made as a thick and filling cereal, or thinned as desired with milk or water.

Grain	Cooking Time (in minutes)
Brown rice (use short grain for a creamier cereal; long grain for more texture)	35 to 40
Bulgur (or cracked wheat)	35 to 40
Cream of Wheat (combine with equal parts wheat germ to boost nutrient value of this refined cereal)	15 to 20
Millet and rolled oats	15 to 20
Stone-ground polenta (or stone-ground corn meal)	20 to 25
Whole wheat couscous	5 to 10

Serve with any combination of toppings

- Fresh fruit or fruit puree
- Milk and brown sugar
- Raisins, honey, nuts
- Honey, sunflower seeds, sun-dried raisins

- Pure maple syrup
- Nut butter with jam/jelly
- Applesauce and/or yogurt
- Bananas, nuts, yogurt

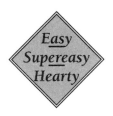

Easy
Supereasy
Hearty

SERVES 1

Simply Fruit (Delicious!)

Bonnie Bruce

I just can't think of anything that's less than great about fruit. For the ultimate in healing and protective nutrients, fruit is simply among the superfoods for snacks, desserts, or even a light meal. Just about all fruits named below are great as they come from nature, whether fresh or dried (except pumpkin, which must be cooked first).

When your digestive tract needs a gentle touch, the good news is that most fruits are also good cooked or stewed and sauced, which helps make them easier to eat and digest. Only a few are best when eaten uncooked (those marked with an asterisk).

Depending on its ripeness, cooked fruit may or may not need some sweetener like honey; add it or not to your own preference.

Don't forget dried fruits, like sun-dried raisins, apricots, peaches and pears, apples, pineapple, mangos, and prunes. These are great high-energy choices when chewing and swallowing are not a problem and your digestive tract is functioning normally. They can also be cooked and pureed for ease in eating and digestion.

Try experimenting and combining different fruits, like peaches with pears or nectarines with blueberries.

PER ½-CUP
SERVING*
*Calories: 50 to 80
Dietary fiber:
varies widely
Protein:
1 to 3 grams
Carbohydrates:
about 15 grams
Good fats: <1 gram
Other fats: <1 gram*

────

**Nutritional value
will vary widely.
Avocado will give
you about 14 grams
of fat (mostly good
fats) per ½ avocado.*

TO COOK OR STEW

Allow 1 piece or ½ cup cut up fruit per serving. Remove any seeds and stems, and peel, if needed. Add a small amount of water to pan and simmer over low heat to desired tenderness. Season with honey, maple syrup, or brown sugar, if desired.

FOR SAUCE

Cook fruit first as above. Then puree in blender or food processor, adding some of the cooking water or some juice as needed.

A Few Favorites

Apples*
Apricots, Peaches
Avocados*
Bananas
Berries (Strawberries,
    Blueberries,
    Blackberries, etc.)
Cherries
Dates

Guavas, Kumquats,
    Passion Fruits,
    Kiwifruits
Figs
Grapefruit*
Grapes*
Mangos
Melons
Nectarines
Oranges*

Papayas
Pears
Persimmons
Pineapples
Plums, prunes
Pumpkin (needs
    sweetener)
Sun-dried raisins
Tangerines*

*Best eaten uncooked.

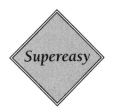

Supereasy

SERVES 4

Fruit Whip with Ricotta Cheese

Bonnie Bruce

Visually appealing with a beautiful orange color from the apricots, this creamy snack or dessert can also be made with peaches. Stir in some cold milk with the ricotta cheese to thin, if you'd like something that's sippable.

2 ripe, medium-size Bartlett pears, peeled, cored, and chopped
1 cup dried apricots
1 two-inch stick cinnamon
1 tablespoon honey
½ cup part-skim ricotta cheese

1. Combine the pears, dried apricots, cinnamon stick, honey, and ½ cup water in a small saucepan. Bring to a boil, then reduce heat. Cover and simmer for 10 to 15 minutes or until fruit is tender.

2. Let fruit mixture cool slightly. Remove cinnamon stick. Blend or process until desired texture. Add ricotta cheese and continue to blend until well mixed.

3. Serve chilled or at room temperature. Keep covered and refrigerated.

PER SERVING
Calories: 149
Dietary fiber:
4 grams
Protein: 5 grams
Carbohydrates:
30 grams
Good fats: 1 gram
Other fats: <1 gram

Whole Wheat Couscous with Dates

Bonnie Bruce

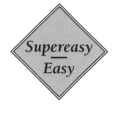

Couscous is a mild flavored traditional North African food made from precooked and dried semolina wheat. Unlike most refined grains, though, plain couscous is not enriched with B vitamins and iron. Be sure to use couscous made from whole wheat, so you'll get the abundance of nutrients found naturally in the whole grain kernel. Couscous cooks up quickly and can be thinned with milk or juice for easier eating and swallowing.

SERVES 2 TO 4

½ cup pitted, chopped dates
1 cup uncooked whole wheat couscous
¼ cup nonfat dry milk powder
2 tablespoons honey
Salt to taste

1. Measure 1¾ cups water into a 2-quart saucepan. Add dates and bring to a boil.
2. Stir couscous and milk powder into boiling water. Cover and remove from heat. Let sit for 5 minutes. Fluff with a fork. Stir in honey, adding more if desired. Salt to taste.

VARIATION

Use different kinds of dried fruit, like sun-dried raisins, chopped dried apricots, or peaches.

PER ¼ RECIPE
Calories: 296
Dietary fiber:
4 grams
Protein: 8 grams
Carbohydrates:
66 grams
Good fats: <1 gram
Other fats: <1 gram

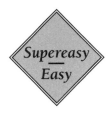

Supereasy
—
Easy

Polenta with Pignolias and Sun-Dried Raisins

Bonnie Bruce

SERVES 3 TO 4

Polenta is a traditional staple food for many Europeans. Usually made from refined coarse cornmeal, we recommend that you use the stone-ground version to get all the beneficial nutrients found naturally in the unrefined grain kernel. This particular recipe is a great snack as well as a light meal, and it reheats very well in the microwave.

¼ cup pignolias (pine nuts), raw or toasted
⅓ cup sun-dried raisins or mixture of other chopped dried
    fruit
1 cup dry stone-ground polenta or stone-ground coarse whole
    grain cornmeal
¼ cup nonfat dry milk powder
2 tablespoons pure maple syrup
Salt to taste

1. Bring 1¾ cups water, pignolias, and raisins to a boil. Then stir in polenta and cook gently until thick, stirring constantly. This should take about 10 minutes.

2. Remove from heat. Cover and let sit for 5 minutes.

3. Stir in milk powder and maple syrup, adding more if desired. Season to taste with salt.

PER ¼ RECIPE
Calories: 223
Dietary fiber:
3 grams
Protein: 6 grams
Carbohydrates:
43 grams
Good fats: 3 grams
Other fats: <1 gram

VARIATION

For a simply wholesome sweet grain dish that's supereasy to eat, omit the pignolias and dried fruit. Thin to desired consistency with milk or water.

Quick 'n' Easy
Fresh Fruit and Yogurt

Bonnie Bruce

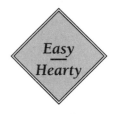

SERVES 1

Quick 'n' easy and very versatile, any kind of fruit works well here. Take advantage of fresh fruit when it is in season. And treat yourself, especially when you're not feeling well, to something special—like beautiful red strawberries in January. Go on, you're worth it!

½ ripe, medium-size banana, sliced

½ cup plain nonfat or lowfat yogurt without gelatin or thickeners

1 tablespoon (or to taste) honey or pure maple syrup

2 tablespoons blanched sliced almonds or chopped walnuts (optional)

Slice banana into bowl. Spoon yogurt over banana. Top with honey or syrup and nuts, if desired.

VARIATION

For an added phytochemical boost, gently mix a tablespoon of wheat germ into the yogurt before adding it to the fruit.

PER SERVING*
Calories: 275
Dietary fiber:
2 grams
Protein: 10 grams
Carbohydrates:
43 grams
Good fats: 6 grams
Other fat: 1 gram

---

*Made with nonfat yogurt and nuts.

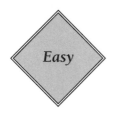

Easy

SERVES 4 TO 6

Rice Pudding with Bananas

Bonnie Bruce

A departure from traditional rice pudding, brown rice and bananas give this wholesome snack or dessert a powerful boost in healthful substances that are vital for your energy and healing needs. Be sure to use short grain brown rice, which gives the pudding its creamy texture.

1 ripe, medium-size banana, sliced
1 tablespoon fresh squeezed lemon juice
2 cups cooked short grain brown rice
¼ cup sun-dried raisins
2 large whole eggs
1 cup nonfat or 1% lowfat milk
¼ cup nonfat dry milk powder
1 teaspoon pure vanilla extract
2 tablespoons honey
½ teaspoon cinnamon
½ cup plain nonfat or lowfat yogurt without gelatin or thickeners

1. Preheat oven to 350 degrees. Gently toss banana with lemon juice to prevent browning. Then spread slices on the bottom of a lightly oiled 8-inch baking dish.

2. Spread cooked rice over banana slices. Sprinkle raisins evenly over the top of the rice.

3. In a blender, whirl eggs, milk, dry milk powder, vanilla, honey, and cinnamon until well mixed. Pour over rice.

4. Bake for 30 minutes. Remove from oven, even though mixture will not be set completely. It will set as it cools. Wait at least 10 minutes, then spread yogurt over top before serving.

VARIATION

If you prefer an easier-to-digest version, cooked short grain white rice can be substituted.

PER ¼ RECIPE*
Calories: 271
Dietary fiber:
3 grams
Protein: 10 grams
Carbohydrates:
51 grams
Good fats: 2 grams
Other fats: 1 gram

*Made with nonfat milk.

Nectarines and Berries
with Yogurt Cheese

Bonnie Bruce

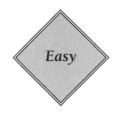

Easy

This is an incredibly simple, appetizing, hi-protein, and easy-to-fix dessert or snack. The juiciness and freshness of the nectarines and berries complement the creaminess of the yogurt cheese. Use any kind of fresh berries or combine different ones (like strawberries with blueberries).

SERVES 3 TO 4

2 cups nonfat or lowfat Yogurt Cheese (page 210)
2 ripe nectarines, peeled and sliced
2 cups fresh ripe berries (such as blueberries or strawberries)
Honey or dark brown sugar to taste

Scoop chilled Yogurt Cheese into a serving dish. Arrange fruit slices artfully around the cheese. Drizzle with honey or sprinkle brown sugar over the fruit for added sweetness.

VARIATIONS

• Part-skim ricotta cheese may be substituted for the Yogurt Cheese, if a milder flavor is preferred.

• For a crunchy touch, try sprinkling pine nuts or other nuts over the cheese and fruit.

• Try other kinds of fruit or fruit sauce (page 209).

PER ¼ RECIPE*
Calories: 160
Dietary fiber:
3 grams
Protein: 10 grams
Carbohydrates:
30 grams
Good fats: <1 gram
Other fats: <1 gram

---

*Made with nonfat Yogurt Cheese.

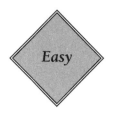

Easy

SERVES 1

Sweet Cooked Apple

Bonnie Bruce

Microwaving is a short cut way to have a wholesome and fresh cooked, traditionally baked apple that is full of flavor and health-giving nutrients. Pears also microwave very nicely this way, but need only about 2 minutes in the microwave. For an easier-to-digest version, peel the fruit and omit the raisins and nuts.

1 baking apple (like Granny Smith), cored and peeled, if desired, and left whole
1 tablespoon sun-dried raisins
1 tablespoon chopped walnuts
1 to 2 teaspoons honey
¼ teaspoon cinnamon
Plain nonfat or lowfat yogurt without gelatin or thickeners for topping (optional)

1. Place apple in microwaveable dish or custard cup. Fill cavity of apple with raisins, walnuts, honey, and cinnamon.

2. Cover with microwave-proof plastic wrap, leaving a small air hole. Cook at full power 3 to 4 minutes or until apple is cooked to desired tenderness. Handle carefully when removing from oven as the cooking bowl may be hot. Serve topped with yogurt, if desired.

PER SERVING*
Calories: 232
Dietary fiber:
3 grams
Protein: 2 grams
Carbohydrates:
47 grams
Good fats: 4 grams
Other fats: <1 gram

———
**Made with raisins
and walnuts.*

Baked Pears and Peaches with Ginger

Bonnie Bruce

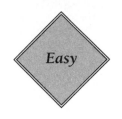

Easy

SERVES 3 TO 4

The ginger in this recipe lends a gentle snap to the richness of these two fruits. For convenience, you can make this soft textured baked fruit dish ahead of time. Keep it in the refrigerator and reheat it or eat it cold. If you are having difficulties chewing or swallowing, omit the walnuts and puree after cooking.

½ cup dried peach halves, chopped
1½ cups ripe but firm Bartlett pears, cored and cut into ½-inch
    slices (peel, if desired)
2 tablespoons sun-dried raisins
1 teaspoon finely grated fresh ginger
1 tablespoon fresh squeezed lemon juice
¼ cup pure maple syrup
½ cup chopped walnuts (optional)

1. Preheat oven to 350 degrees. In a medium bowl, combine dried peaches, pear slices, raisins, ginger, lemon juice, syrup, and walnuts. Gently toss to mix well.

2. Place in single layer on nonstick or lightly oiled baking sheet. Bake for 10 to 15 minutes, or until done to desired consistency.

VARIATION

Add nectarines and thinly sliced apples for a delightful fruit medley.

PER ¼ RECIPE*
*Calories: 192
Dietary fiber:
4 grams
Protein: 1 gram
Carbohydrates:
46 grams
Good fats: <1 gram
Total fat: <1 gram*

*Made without
walnuts.*

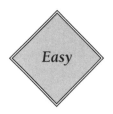

Easy

SERVES 4

Vanilla Pears with Strawberries

Bonnie Bruce

Fresh pears embellished by a light poaching in a mild honey vanilla sauce are complemented by the sweet-tart flavor of strawberries. Turn this into a light brunch time meal by serving it with part-skim ricotta cheese.

4 ripe but firm Bartlett pears, peeled, cored, and halved
3 tablespoons fresh squeezed lemon juice
½ cup mild honey
1 vanilla bean, slit lengthwise (1 teaspoon pure vanilla extract may be substituted)
3 strips orange peel, ½-inch long each
1 cup fresh strawberry halves
Plain yogurt and mint leaves for garnish

1. Rub pear halves with lemon juice to prevent browning and set aside.

2. In a pan large enough to hold the pear halves in a single layer, combine 1¾ cups of water, honey, vanilla bean or vanilla extract, and orange peel. Bring mixture to a boil, being careful not to let it boil over. Lower heat.

3. Place pears in the pan, flat side down. Simmer gently for 3 to 5 minutes, or until fruit is just barely tender. Then slide strawberry halves into the hot liquid with the pears only long enough to heat (less than 1 minute). Do not let strawberries cook.

4. Remove pears and strawberries from the pan with a slotted spoon. Place 2 pear halves on each dish. Arrange strawberries attractively around pears. Drizzle cooking liquid over top, if desired. Serve with a dollop of plain yogurt and garnish with mint leaves.

PER SERVING
Calories: 188
Dietary fiber:
5 grams
Protein: 1 gram
Carbohydrates:
46 grams
Good fats: <1 gram
Other fats: <1 gram

VARIATIONS

• Use fresh peaches or nectarines instead of pears (note that cooking time may need to be shortened).

• Sprinkle finely chopped almonds over the top before serving.

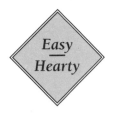

Bread Pudding of the Ancients

Bonnie Bruce

In days of old, when whole grains were in the majority and white flour was uncommon, baked goods were naturally full of disease-fighting nutrients. This traditional recipe takes you back to those times, as its main ingredient is whole grain bread. Vary the kind of bread from those with seeds or nuts to those made from different kinds of grains. You may wish to start with 100 percent whole wheat, which is softer in texture than breads with nuts and seeds. The walnuts may also be omitted for easier digestion.

4 slices whole grain bread, diced or torn into small pieces (day old or stale bread works well here)
⅓ cup sun-dried raisins or other chopped dried fruit as desired
½ cup chopped walnuts (optional)
2 cups nonfat or 1% lowfat milk
¼ cup dry nonfat milk powder
2 large whole eggs
¼ teaspoon salt
½ teaspoon cinnamon
¼ teaspoon freshly grated nutmeg
2 teaspoons pure vanilla extract
3 tablespoons honey

PER ¼ RECIPE
Calories: 377
Dietary fiber:
3 grams
Protein: 15 grams
Carbohydrates:
50 grams
Good fats: 11 grams
Other fats: 2 grams

*Made with nonfat milk and walnuts.

1. Preheat oven to 350 degrees. Lightly oil a 9-inch baking pan. Line bottom of pan with bread pieces. Then top with raisins and nuts, if using.

2. In a bowl or blender, mix together the milk, milk powder, eggs, salt, cinnamon, nutmeg, vanilla, and honey. Pour into

pan and make sure that all the bread is coated with the liquid mixture.

3. Bake for 25 to 30 minutes or until knife inserted into center comes out clean. Great to eat warm or cold.

VARIATION

Substitute different kinds of dried fruits, like dried apricots or peaches, for the raisins.

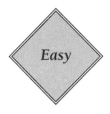

Easy

SERVES 4 TO 6

Apple Bake with a Hint of Maple

Bonnie Bruce

Made from simple and pure ingredients, this recipe maximizes the nutritional benefits of fruit. As a sweet ending to a meal or a snappy way to start the day, this delicious apple crisp-like dish is sure to be appealing. We've left the peel on the apples to add fiber; but if you'd like something easier to eat and digest, they can be peeled before cooking.

4 ripe medium-size Granny Smith apples, cored and cut into
   ¼-inch slices
1 tablespoon fresh squeezed lemon juice
⅓ cup sun-dried raisins
4 teaspoons tapioca
4 tablespoons pure maple syrup
½ cup rolled oats
¼ cup honey
1 to 2 tablespoons almond butter

1. Preheat oven to 350 degrees. Lightly oil an 8-inch square or round baking dish. In a bowl, toss apples with lemon juice to prevent them from browning.

2. Turn the apples into the baking dish and press the slices down. Sprinkle raisins and tapioca over apples. Then pour syrup and 2 tablespoons water over them.

PER ¼ RECIPE
Calories: 259
Dietary fiber:
4 grams
Protein: 3 grams
Carbohydrates:
55 grams
Good fat: 3 grams
Other fats: <1 gram

3. Prepare topping by combining oats, honey, and almond butter together. Spread over top of apples, trying to cover as much of the apples as possible.

4. Cover with foil and bake for 25 to 30 minutes. Remove foil and continue baking until apples are tender, about 10 minutes more. If the topping begins to brown too much, recover with foil during the last 5 to 10 minutes of baking.

Chapter 15

BASIC BUT ESSENTIAL

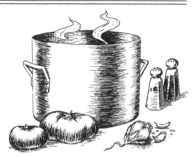

BASIC AND ESSENTIAL RECIPES ARE THE ONES THAT CON-tribute special touches to meals, either by accompanying them, enhancing them, or becoming an integral part of a recipe. They vary from sweet to savory, and none is very difficult to prepare.

For example, the Simple Vegetable Stock perks up the flavor of any soup in place of water, while also enriching it with numerous health-enhancing compounds. Simply Perfect Tomato Sauce will turn plain pasta, rice, or even fresh cooked vegetables into a quick and flavorful meal that will perk up everyday fare. And you'll find that the high-protein, easily digested Yogurt Cheese is a food that complements fruit, whole grain bread, and vegeta-bles—or is just as good by itself. Nature's Own Fruit Sauce 'n' Spread brings you a delightful, winning fruit flavor to dress yogurt, ricotta, or cottage cheese and bread.

Pointers for Basic But Essential recipes:

• Some of the recipes are excellent as make-ahead items to store for when you're not feeling well. The Simple Vegetable Stock and the Simply Perfect Tomato Sauce freeze very well and can be kept for several weeks. Try freezing them in ice cube trays and then add the frozen "flavor cubes" to recipes of your choice.

• Vary the Simply Perfect Tomato Sauce by changing the herbs; for example, use oregano and rosemary instead of or in addition to the basil.

• Make the Simple Vegetable Stock more robust by adding different root vegetables, like potatoes and rutabagas, or different kinds of onions.

Basic but Essential

Supereasy recipes are smooth sippable foods for ease in swallowing without need to chew.

Easy recipes are soft and tender, need some chewing but are gentle on the digestive tract.

Hearty recipes are most suitable when you are feeling well and back to normal.

Recipe	Supereasy	Easy	Hearty
Simple Vegetable Stock (*page 207*)	◆		
Simply Perfect Tomato Sauce (*page 208*)	◆		
Nature's Own Fruit Sauce 'n' Spread (*page 209*)	◆		
Yogurt Cheese (*page 210*)		◆	
Baked Garlic (*page 211*)	◆		
Creamy Garbanzo Spread (*page 212*)	◆	◆	◆

Simple Vegetable Stock

Bonnie Bruce

Supereasy

MAKES ABOUT
2½ QUARTS

This stock adds flavor to any soup or stew, is fairly easy to prepare, and freezes well. Freeze it in ice cube trays to make "flavor cubes" and use by dropping them into a soup as it cooks (each cube is about two tablespoons). Instead of discarding the cooked vegetables, try pureeing and using them to thicken or flavor other recipes. If you use wine, there will be a small amount of alcohol remaining even after cooking the stock. Feel free to omit it if you prefer.

1 tablespoon extra virgin olive oil
3 celery stalks with leaves, cut into 1-inch slices
3 carrots, cut into 1-inch slices
1 large onion, chopped
3 cloves garlic, peeled and left whole
¼ cup chopped fresh Italian parsley
1 bay leaf
1 teaspoon dried thyme leaves
1 cup white wine (optional)
1 tablespoon miso (optional)
Salt and freshly ground pepper

1. Gently warm the oil in a large 4- to 6-quart soup kettle. Add the celery, carrots, onion, garlic, parsley, bay leaf, and thyme. Cover and cook over low heat, stirring occasionally, until vegetables are tender (about 15 to 20 minutes).

2. Add 3 quarts of water and the wine (if using). Bring to a boil, then simmer uncovered for an hour. Remove bay leaf. Mix miso (if using) with 2 tablespoons water and stir into the stock. Strain vegetables. Season to taste with salt and pepper.

3. Stock is ready. If freezing, let cool slightly then pour into containers or ice cube trays.

PER CUP*
Calories: 29
Dietary fiber:
1 gram
Protein: <1 gram
Carbohydrates:
5 grams
Good fats: 1 gram
Other fats: <1 gram
_____
*Made with wine
and miso.

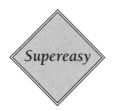

Supereasy

MAKES ABOUT
6 CUPS

Simply Perfect Tomato Sauce

Bonnie Bruce

This is a sauce of many uses that is chock full of healthful phyto-chemicals (see page 11). It's easy to make, freezes well, and makes a quick topping for pasta, polenta, or even tofu cubes. It purees into a very nice creamy sauce if you prefer something smooth.

1 tablespoon extra virgin olive oil
1 to 2 cloves garlic, peeled and chopped
6 to 8 cups fresh ripe, medium-size tomatoes, peeled if
    desired, and chopped (do not puree, chunks are important to
    texture) or a 28-ounce can of good quality tomatoes,
    chopped and drained
1 cup chopped fresh basil leaves
Salt and freshly ground pepper

1. Gently warm the oil in a medium saucepan. Cook garlic over low to moderate heat for 2 to 3 minutes or until just barely tender without letting it brown.

2. Add tomatoes and basil. Bring to a boil. Then lower heat and simmer for 20 to 30 minutes. Season to taste with salt and pepper. Spoon over hot pasta or grains and serve immediately.

VARIATION

PER CUP
Calories: 74
Dietary fiber:
3 grams
Protein: 2 grams
Carbohydrates:
12 grams
Good fats: 2 grams
Other fats: <1 gram

Add a cup of sliced mushrooms with the tomatoes and basil.

Nature's Own Fruit Sauce 'n' Spread

Bonnie Bruce

Supereasy

MAKES 2 TO 3
CUPS

This recipe lends itself to a wide variety of fresh fruit. Make it with fruit that is ripe and in season whenever you can. Try it on top of plain yogurt or part-skim ricotta cheese. As a spread, it may be softer than you're used to, but it spreads very smoothly and tastes great on whole grain bread with nut butter. For a sweet treat, it can even be eaten by itself with a spoon. For a very digestible spread, strain out any seeds before serving.

2 cups finely chopped or pureed unsweetened fresh
   strawberries
¼ cup fresh squeezed orange juice or other juice of choice
3 to 4 tablespoons honey
1½ tablespoons arrowroot
Pinch of nutmeg or cinnamon (optional)

1. Place fruit (chopped or pureed) in medium saucepan with the orange juice and honey. Bring to a low boil and cook, stirring regularly, for about 2 to 3 minutes or until fruit reaches desired doneness.

2. While the fruit is cooking, dissolve arrowroot in 2 tablespoons water. Then stir it into the fruit. Reduce heat to low. Continue to simmer over very low heat until mixture thickens.

3. Remove from heat and store refrigerated in covered jar. Keeps for about a week.

VARIATION

Try blueberries, raspberries, or any other berries as desired. Peeled, chopped peaches, nectarines, plums, and apricots also work very well.

PER ½ CUP
Calories: 56
Dietary fiber:
1 gram
Protein: <1 gram
Carbohydrates:
14 grams
Good fats: <1 gram
Other fats: <1 gram

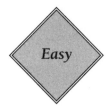

Easy

MAKES ABOUT
2 CUPS

Yogurt Cheese

Bonnie Bruce

This centuries old recipe is quite versatile and can be used for desserts, as well as stirred into soups or added to pureed vegetables such as mashed potatoes for added protein. For dessert, try it with fresh fruit or fruit purees (such as Nature's Own Fruit Sauce 'n' Spread on page 209). Yogurt Cheese is incredibly easy to make once you do the simple preparation; it literally makes itself overnight. For the best and most nourishing results, use yogurt without added gelatin or thickeners.

> 4 cups (1 quart) plain nonfat or lowfat yogurt without gelatin
>   or thickeners

1. Wet a cheesecloth by running it under cold water and squeezing out the excess liquid. Line a strainer with a double layer of the cheesecloth. Place the strainer in a bigger bowl that will keep the yogurt from sitting in the whey as it drains out. The whey is a protein-rich liquid that drains from the yogurt. You can use it in soups, to cook vegetables, or to drink as is. The yellowish color and the taste of it, though, make it sometimes unappealing as a beverage by itself to some people.

2. Spoon or pour the yogurt into the cheesecloth-lined strainer. Then fold the ends of the cheesecloth over the top of the yogurt. Refrigerate yogurt in the strainer, uncovered, and leave overnight.

3. The next day, check the thickness of the yogurt. When it is the consistency you desire, remove it from the strainer. The longer you let it drain, the more solid it will become. Store refrigerated in sealed container. Keeps for about two weeks.

PER ½ CUP*
Calories: 132
Dietary fiber:
<1 gram
Protein: 14 grams
Carbohydrates:
19 grams
Good fats: <1 gram
Other fats: <1 gram

Made with nonfat yogurt.

Baked Garlic

Bonnie Bruce

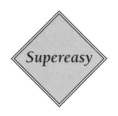

Supereasy

MAKES 4
HEADS

Baking garlic gives it a soft, mild flavor and a creamy texture. It is very easy to make and adds a special finish and valuable cancer-fighting substances to soups, salad dressings, vegetables, or when you simply spread it on bread.

4 large heads garlic
2 tablespoons extra virgin olive oil

1. Preheat oven to 400 degrees. Rub excess papery skin off garlic heads without separating cloves. Slice about ½ inch off top of each head.

2. Place the 4 heads on a piece of aluminum foil big enough to make a folded package over them. Drizzle the olive oil over the garlic heads. Pinch the edges of the foil together to make a package.

3. Bake for 40 to 45 minutes or until cloves are very soft. Unwrap and let cool slightly. Store baked garlic in the refrigerator. It keeps for three to four days. If desired, squeeze out garlic puree all at once and keep in a covered jar ready for use.

PER GARLIC
HEAD
Calories: 97
Dietary fiber:
1 gram
Protein: 2 grams
Carbohydrates:
11 grams
Good fats: 5 grams
Other fats: <1 gram

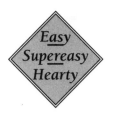

Easy
Supereasy
Hearty

MAKES 1½
CUPS

Creamy Garbanzo Spread

Bonnie Bruce

This mild-flavored spread complements soft whole grain bread or it can be used to top a baked potato for a light main dish. It can be thinned for easier swallowing, as desired, by adding a little water. For the greatest nutritional punch, we recommend that fresh, cooked garbanzo beans be used. Canned beans may be used, but the flavor will be slightly different, and the spread will be higher in sodium.

1¾ cups cooked garbanzo beans
¼ cup sesame butter (tahini)
2 tablespoons fresh squeezed lemon juice
1 large clove garlic, peeled and left whole
¼ teaspoon cumin powder
Salt and freshly ground pepper to taste

Put all ingredients into a food processor bowl. Process to desired texture. Add a tablespoon or two of water if you would like a smoother or thinner spread. Season to taste with salt and pepper.

VARIATIONS

• To make this recipe Supereasy, put the beans through a ricer to remove the skins before combining with other ingredients.
• For a lighter version of the spread, omit the sesame butter.
• Try it as a dip for fresh vegetables.

PER ¼ CUP
Calories: 129
Dietary fiber:
3 grams
Protein: 6 grams
Carbohydrates:
15 grams
Good fats: 5 grams
Other fats: <1 gram

Recipes That Freeze Well

With a little care, frozen foods can provide delicious nourishment on days when you don't feel up to cooking. Some tips for freezing:

• Freeze leftovers and extra batches of recipes in single-serving containers for quick, easy meals. In general, the recipes below should keep well in the freezer for up to two months.

• Remember to label each container with the name of the food and the date you froze it.

• To maintain food quality, be sure that the container is covered or sealed tightly.

• When heating in the microwave, follow your oven manufacturer's directions for cooking frozen foods.

• When heating in a conventional oven, thaw your food in the refrigerator to reduce chances of bacterial growth (which can happen if food is thawed at room temperature). Cooked foods should be kept at room temperature or in the refrigerator only for very short amounts of time.

RECIPES TO FREEZE

Apple Bake with a Hint of Maple *(page 204)*
Apricot-Mango Frozen Yogurt Smoothie *(page 88)*
Barley and Friends *(page 128)*

Broccoli Bisque *(page 117)*
Brown Rice Pilaf with Apples and Sun-Dried Raisins *(page 150)*
Creamy Potato and Yam Soup *(page 111)*
Dilled Carrot and Yam Soup *(page 116)*
Golden Red Lentil Soup *(page 123)*
Harvest Squash and Apple Soup *(page 114)*
Juice Cubies *(page 86)*
Medley of Rices with Pumpkin Seeds *(page 154)*
Millet and Carrot Pilaf *(page 138)*
Peachy Lemon Smoothie *(page 94)*
Potato Puree with Baked Garlic *(page 171)*
Potato Soup with Spinach Ribbons *(page 122)*
Puree of Fresh Fennel *(page 112)*
Ragout of Brown Rice, Yams, Tomatoes, and Beans *(page 155)*
Raspberry Kefir Smoothie *(page 92)*
Red Lentil Soup with Fresh Greens *(page 125)*
Simple Vegetable Stock *(page 207)*
Simply Perfect Tomato Sauce *(page 208)*
Simply Squash *(page 172)*
Whole Wheat Couscous with Mushrooms *(page 136)*
Ziti and Cannellini Hot Pot *(page 126)*

Rate Your Way of Eating: How Well Has It Been Working for You?

Here are some key questions that will give you an idea of whether or not your past diet maximized all the possible healing and protective factors from foods. Answer yes or no to each question as it applied to your typical diet before you started treatment or were feeling ill.

DAILY

Whole grain foods   Did you eat at least *6 servings* (1 serving = 1 slice or ½ cup cooked), such as whole grain breads (made with whole wheat flour as first ingredient listed, not wheat flour), hulled barley (not pearled), brown rice, bulgur or cracked wheat, buckwheat, stone-ground cornmeal, whole wheat couscous, millet, oats, whole wheat pasta, wheat germ, quinoa, and wild rice?

☐ YES
☐ NO

Orange or red vegetables or fruits (fresh, dried, or cooked) Did you eat at least *2 servings* (1 serving = 1/2 cup or 1 medium piece), such as carrots, tomatoes, red bell peppers, oranges, winter squash, pumpkin, sweet potatoes, apricots, peaches, nectarines, mangos, papayas, cantaloupe, berries, and their natural juices?

☐ YES
☐ NO

Dark green and leafy green vegetables Did you eat at least *1 serving* (1 serving = ½ cup cooked or 1 cup raw), such as green peppers, broccoli, green cabbage, spinach, Swiss chard, kale, collards, mustard or turnip greens, sprouts, romaine lettuce and other leafy salad greens, or a mixture of any of these? (Do not count iceberg lettuce.)

YES ☐
NO ☐

Other vegetables or fruits Did you eat at least *1 serving* (1 serving = ½ cup or 1 medium piece), such as potatoes, green beans, cucumbers, asparagus, avocados, figs, grapes, apples, bananas, pears, etc.? (Do not include fried vegetables like french fries.)

YES ☐
NO ☐

Nonfat or lowfat dairy products Did you eat at least *2 servings* (1 serving = approximately 1 cup), such as nonfat or lowfat milk, yogurt, kefir, buttermilk, part-skim ricotta, or cottage cheese?

YES ☐
NO ☐

YES ☐ NO ☐ *Alcohol* Did you have *1 or less drinks* of alcoholic beverages?

ON A WEEKLY BASIS

Cruciferous vegetables Did you eat at least *3 servings* (1 serving = ½ cup), such as broccoli, Brussels sprouts, cauliflower, cabbage, kale, collards, rutabagas, parsnips, and turnips?

YES ☐
NO ☐

YES ☐
NO ☐ *Onions, leeks, shallots, or garlic* Did you include these seasonings in your meals at least *5 or 6 times?*

Legumes, nuts and seeds, and their butters Did you include cooked dry beans (such as white beans, garbanzos, kidneys, pintos or black beans), lentils, split peas, tofu, tempeh, nuts and seeds and their butters (such as almonds, hazelnuts, walnuts, pine nuts, sunflower seeds, tahini, or peanut butter) at least *4 times?*

YES ☐
NO ☐

Extra virgin olive oil, sesame oil, and avocado oil   Did you use these oils on salads, vegetables, or in food preparation as your *only fats?*

☐ YES
☐ NO

SCORING

Although these questions may not include all of the foods you ate, they will reveal two things.

1. Each "yes" response indicates where you were doing the best possible to get enough of the healing and protective factors contained in those foods. An eating pattern reflected by "yes" responses helps to ensure that your food choices will work for you during treatment, during recovery, and beyond to protect you from future illness.

2. "No" responses give you some goals to work toward to optimize your intake of all the goodness nature has to offer.

APPENDIX C

Stocking Your Pantry

Keeping a well-stocked pantry gives you freedom and variety to prepare good, wholesome food at any time of the day or night, whenever you get the whim. Make photocopies of this and use it as a shopping list.

Pantry staples to keep on hand	Refrigerator staples
Whole Grains and Cereals	*General*
Barley (best: hulled)	Eggs
Brown rice (short and long grain)	Fresh juices/nectars
Buckwheat	Nonfat or 1% lowfat milk
Bulgur or cracked wheat	Miso
Couscous (best: whole wheat)	Part skim ricotta cheese
Millet	Nonfat or lowfat cottage cheese
Oats	Tempeh
Pasta (best: made from whole wheat or	Tofu
100% durum wheat semolina flour)	Nonfat or lowfat yogurt without
Stone-ground cornmeal	thickeners and gelatins
Wheat germ	Fresh ginger root
Wild rice	
	Some Fruits and Vegetables
	That Keep Well
Fruits and Vegetables	
Canned cooked beans	Citrus fruits (oranges, lemons)
Canned tomatoes (good quality)	Apples
Dry beans, lentils, and split peas	Pears
Garlic	Grapes
Nut butters (best: without added	Bananas
artificial fats or sugars)	Carrots

Pantry staples to keep on hand	Refrigerator staples
Onions	Celery
Potatoes	Winter squash (hard shelled)
Seeds (sesame, sunflower)	
Sun-dried raisins	Other items that I need:
Dried apricots	_____
Dried peaches, pineapple, etc.	_____
Whole nuts (almonds, walnuts, pine nuts, hazelnuts, etc.)	_____
Rutabagas, turnips, parsnips	_____
	_____

Condiments

Extra virgin olive oil
Wheat germ oil
Sesame Oil
Pure maple syrup
Honey
Pure vanilla extract and other natural
   flavorings (like lemon)
Nonfat dry milk powder
Dried herbs and spices
Vinegars
Pepper
Sea salt
Soy and tamari sauces
Blackstrap molasses

Safe Food Handling and Storage

No kitchen pantry can be healthful if it isn't safe. The last thing we want to do is become ill from not handling food safely. Important always, but especially if the immune system is low, proper food storage is essential to keeping your food safe. The storage guidelines below are based on "ideal" conditions and temperatures. Proper temperature for refrigerator storage is 40° to 60° F (4° to 16° C). Remember: Never try even one bite of a food that you suspect might have gone bad.

About Keeping Cooked Foods

Always chill them as soon as possible after eating. Don't keep cooked foods at room temperature for more than two hours. If you find that you can only tolerate or only want to eat warm or room temperature foods, try to limit the amount of time foods are left out.

About Storing Leftovers

Leftovers are great to have on hand. Be sure to store them (or planned extra food) in clean plastic, glass, ceramic, or stainless steel containers to avoid contamination by bacteria or other substances. Cover securely and store properly in the freezer or refrigerator.

Grains and Legumes

Uncooked grains   In general, for immediate use and short term storage (like a few weeks to a month), store covered in a dark, cool cupboard.

Whole grains   If your kitchen gets rather warm, keep them in the refrigerator to prevent development of pests. Otherwise, store in sealed containers in a cool, dark cupboard. They should keep for several months.

Dried pastas and rice   These will keep for at least a year in a cool place. They tend to be quite resistant to infestation.

Whole grain breads   Store tightly wrapped in the refrigerator or at room temperature for one to three days. They can be frozen for about a year. Whole grain breads without preservatives and additives tend to become stale or moldy within a few days. Discard if any sign of mold occurs.

Cooked grains and beans   Store covered in the refrigerator up to seven days. Freeze if longer storage time is desired.

Uncooked dry beans   Store in tightly closed container in cool, dark place. Most generally have a keeping time of at least a year.

Tofu and tempeh   Keep refrigerated. Note the expiration date on the package. If you use only a portion of the package, note that tofu especially will tend to perish rapidly after being opened. Store opened tofu in the refrigerator in a covered bowl filled with water.

Nuts, seeds, and their butters   Store in an airtight container. Most will keep from 6 to 12 months. If there is any sign of mold, discard immediately.

Fruits and Vegetables

Fresh fruits   Most can be kept at room temperature to ripen and then should be refrigerated. Keeping time at room temperature varies widely depending upon the variety. For example, apples and most citrus fruits tend to have a longer keeping time than ripe peaches. Discard if any signs of deterioration or spoilage occur.

Dried fruit   Store tightly covered in a dark, cool cupboard. Dried fruits usually have a relatively long, although variable, shelf-life. Discard if any mold or deterioration occurs.

Juices and nectars   Keep covered in the refrigerator. Storage time will vary depending on the fruit and freshness of the squeezing. Best bet is to use fresh squeezed, especially within a few days.

Fresh vegetables   Keep most varieties, except for tomatoes and some root vegetables (like potatoes and onions) refrigerated. Keeping times vary widely depending on freshness—from a day to several weeks—with root vegetables usually having the longest life.

Cooked fruits and vegetables   Keep covered in the refrigerator for five to seven days. Discard if there is any change in color, texture, or smell.

Oils

Oils   Store in a dark or cool place such as the refrigerator. Harmless clouding may occur when refrigerated.

Miscellaneous

Miso   Keep well covered or wrapped for a few months. Store refrigerated, unless it's the dry variety.

Sweeteners

• Honey: Store in a covered container. Honey has a variable life span. If it becomes granulated, it is still good. A gentle heating over a double boiler will help dissolve sugar crystals that have formed.

• Pure maple syrup: Store covered in a cool spot or refrigerator. Pure maple syrup also has a variable life span.

• Molasses: Store in a covered container. It has a variable life span, but generally lasts several months.

Herbs and spices   Keep dried herbs and spices in airtight containers and out of direct light; most will keep for about six months (after that they tend to lose flavor). Keep fresh herbs covered in the refrigerator. Most are best when used within a few days.

Animal Foods

Yogurt, ricotta, and cottage cheese   Keep covered and refrigerated for up to two weeks. Discard immediately if any sign of odor or discoloration is detected.

Nonfat milk   Store refrigerated in an opaque, tightly closed container for up to a week.

Eggs   Keep covered and refrigerated in original carton for up to two weeks.

APPENDIX E

Shopping Sources

WHOLE GRAINS,
WHOLE GRAIN FLOURS,
AND BEANS

Arrowhead Mills, Inc.
110 South Lawton
Hereford, TX 79045
806-364-0730
Whole grains, whole grain
flours, and beans.

Deer Valley Farms
P.O. Box 173
Guilford, NY 13780

Giusto's Specialty Foods
241 East Harris Avenue
South San Francisco, CA
94080
415-873-6566
Whole grains and whole grain
flours.

Gold Mine Natural Food Co.
3419 Hancock Street
San Diego, CA 92110-4307
800-474-3663
Whole grains, beans, and
kitchen equipment.

Shiloh Farms
P.O. Box 97
Sulphur Springs, AR 72768
Whole grains and whole grain
flour.

Tadco/Niblack
900 Jefferson Road, Building 5
Rochester, NY 14623

Walnut Acres
Penns Creek, PA 17862
717-847-0601
Whole grains and whole grain
flour.

CULTURES FOR MILK, SOY PRODUCTS, AND BREADMAKING

Alton-Spiller, Inc
P.O. 696
Los Altos, CA 94023
Starters and supplies for whole grain bread making.

GEM Cultures
30301 Sherwood Road
Fort Bragg, CA 95437
707-964-2922
Sourdough starters including barm; tempeh, miso, and other cultured soy products; kefir and other unusual milk cultures; sea vegetation and food culturing cookbooks.

Rosell Institute, Inc.
8480 Boulevard St-Laurent
Montréal, Quebec H2P 2M6
Canada
514-381-5631
Cultures for yogurt, kefir, buttermilk, acidophilus milk; insulated yogurt maker.

HERB AND SPICES, PLANTS AND SEEDS

Seeds of Change
621 Old Santa Fe Trail #10
P.O. Box 15700
Santa Fe, NM 87501
505-983-8956

Shepherd's Garden Seeds
6116 Highway 9
Felton, CA 95018
408-335-6945
Both Seeds of Change and Shepherd's Garden Seeds have a wonderful edible flower and herb seed collection to help you get started growing safe flowers and fresh herbs.

KITCHEN EQUIPMENT

Sassafras Enterprises, Inc.
1622 West Carol Avenue
Chicago, IL 60612
312-226-2000
Unglazed ceramic baking tiles, bread cloches (domes), and baking pots.

Williams-Sonoma
100 North Point Street
San Francisco, CA 94133
415-421-7900
Specialty kitchen equipment.

OLIVES AND EXTRA VIRGIN OLIVE OILS

Santa Barbara Olive Co.
P.O. Box 1570
Santa Inez, CA 93460
805-688-9917
Olives and olive oils.

Sadeg
P.O. Box 4014236
Alameda, CA 94501
510-521-6548
California olive oils.

Sciabica
P.O. Box 1246
Modesto, CA 95353
209-577-5067
California olive oils.

The Stutz Company
2600 Tenth Street
Berkeley, CA 94710-2486
510-644-2200
California olive oils.

BROWN RICE

Lundberg Family Farms
P.O. Box 369
Richvale, CA 95974
916-882-4551
Specialty brown rice varieties.

SEA VEGETATION

Mainecoast Sea Vegetables
Shore Road
Franklin, ME 04634
207-565-2907
Edible sea vegetation and
related food products.

Rising Tide Sea Vegetables
P.O. Box 1914
Mendocino, CA 95460
707-937-2109
Edible sea vegetation.

TEAS

Silk Road Teas
P.O. Box 287
Lagunitas, CA 94938
415-488-9017

VEGETABLE OILS

Spectrum Natural
133 Copeland Street
Petaluma, CA 94952
707-778-8900
A wide variety of vegetable
oils.

JUICERS

Vita-Mix Corporation
8615 Usher Road
Cleveland, OH 44138
216-235-4840
High-power blender and
homogenizer.

Plastakat
6220 E. Highway 12
Lodi, CA 95240
209-369-2154
Juicers.

POWDERED MEAL DIETS

Shaklee Corporation
444 Market Street
San Franscisco, CA 94111
415 954-3000

References

Many books and articles were consulted in the writing of this book. Those listed below were particularly helpful.

Ensminger, Audrey, Ensminger, M.E., Konlande, James, and Robson, John. *The Concise Encyclopedia of Foods and Nutrition.* Boca Raton, FL: CRC Press, 1995.

Estella, Mary. *Natural Foods Cookbook: Vegetarian Dairy-Free Cuisine.* Tokyo: Japan Publications Inc., 1985.

Foster, Steven. *Herbal Renaissance.* Salt Lake City: Gibbs Smith, 1984.

Garland, Sarah. *The Complete Book of Herbs and Spices.* New York: Viking, 1979.

Greene, Bert. *The Grains Cookbook.* New York: Workman Publishing Company Inc., 1988.

Harpham, Wendy. *After Cancer: A Guide to Your New Life.* New York: HarperCollins Publishers Inc., 1994.

Kilham, Christopher. *The Bread and Circus Whole Food Bible: How to select and prepare safe healthful foods without pesticides or chemical additives.* Reading, Massachusetts: Addison-Wesley, 1991.

Margen, S. and Editors of the University of California at Berkeley Wellness Letter. *The Wellness Encyclopedia of Food and Nutrition: How to Buy, Store, and Prepare Every Fresh Food.* New York: Random House, 1992.

McGee, Harold. *On Food and Cooking: The Science and Lore of the Kitchen.* New York: Charles Scribner's Sons, 1984.

Moyers, B. *Healing and the Mind.* New York: Doubleday, 1993.

National Cancer Institute. *Eating Hints for Cancer Patients: NIH Pub. #94-2079.* Washington. D.C.: US Dept. of Health and Human Services, 1994.

Owen, Sri. *The Rice Book.* New York: St. Martin's Press, 1993.

Quillin, Patric, Williams, R. Michael (eds.). *Adjuvant Nutrition in Cancer Treatment: 1992 Symposium Proceedings.* Arlington Heights, IL: Cancer Treatment Research Foundation, 1993.

Roden, Claudia. *Mediterranean Cookery.* New York: Alfred A. Knopf, 1987.

Spiller, Gene and Hubbard, Rowena. *Nutrition Secrets of the Ancients.* Rocklin, CA: Prima Publishing, 1996.

Spiller, Gene. *Eat Your Way to Better Health.* Prima Publishing, 1996.

Zeman, Frances and Ney, Denise. *Applications in Medical Nutrition Therapy.* Englewood Cliffs, New Jersey: Prentice-Hall, 1996.

Index